Dr. Jenner
and the
Speckled Monster

D1262370

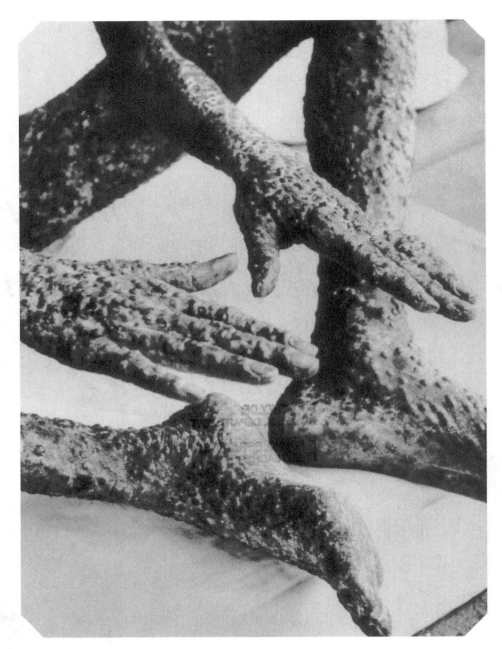

The Speckled Monster rages. In this photograph, taken in Africa in the 1960s, a man's arms and legs, and probably his entire body, are covered with large pustules. The sufferer appears to have a severe case of the disease, and probably did not survive. PHOTO COURTESY OF THE WORLD HEALTH ORGANIZATION

Dr. Jenner and the Speckled Monster

The Search for the Smallpox Vaccine

Albert Marrin

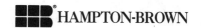 HAMPTON-BROWN

For our good friend, Dr. Stanley Mirsky, a true scientist in the Jennerian tradition

Dr. Jenner and the Speckled Monster by Albert Marrin
Copyright © 2002 by Albert Marrin

Cover Photo Credits:
(background) *Millions of vaccine doses contributed to the success of the worldwide eradication campaign* (World Health Organization); *Portrait of a Killer*, electron microscope photo of smallpox virus, courtesy of Albert Marrin; *Smallpox: Gale, Abcès, et Ulcères; Causés par la Vaccine* and *The hand Jenner used as a source for his vaccine*, by Edward Jenner (National Library of Medicine).

On-Page Coach™ (introductions, questions, on-page glossaries),
The Exchange, back cover summary © Hampton-Brown.

Hampton-Brown
P.O. Box 223220
Carmel, California 93922
800-333-3510
www.hampton-brown.com

Printed in the United States of America

ISBN-13: 0-978-0-7362-3167-1
ISBN-10: 0-7362-3167-6

13 14 15 10 9 8 7 6 5 4 3

Thou shalt not be afraid for the terror by night;
nor for the arrow that flieth by day; nor for
the pestilence that walketh in darkness.

—Psalm 91 : 5–6

"A medical man, from the nature of things,
is always groping like a miner in the dark
without the benefit of a safety lamp."

—Edward Jenner

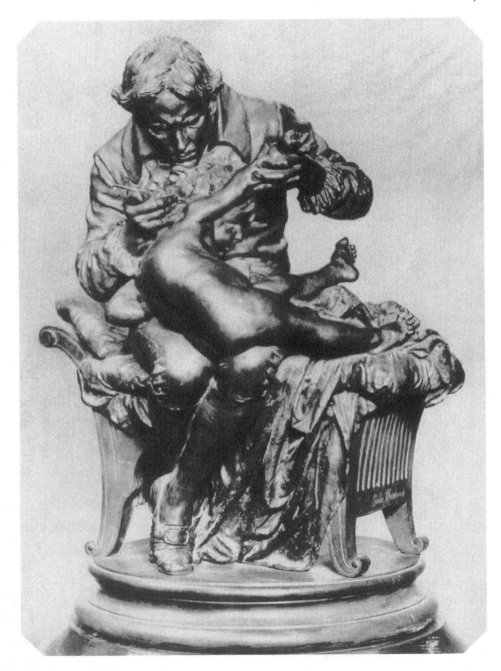

This marble statue, the work of an anonymous Italian sculptor, shows Dr. Jenner vaccinating an infant. PHOTO COURTESY OF THE NATIONAL LIBRARY OF MEDICINE

Table of Contents

*I*ntroduction

Dr. Jenner and the Speckled Monster is about Dr. Jenner's **determined** search for a smallpox vaccine. Before the development of a vaccine, people feared smallpox more than any other disease in history. It struck without warning. It killed millions of people. It blinded many others.

During the eighteenth and nineteenth centuries, people called smallpox the "Speckled Monster." This name described the terrible spots that appeared all over the body. Smallpox spread quickly and easily through the air. During a smallpox **epidemic**, many people died very quickly. Doctors were not able to stop the spread of the disease. Then, all of a sudden, smallpox would disappear for years. But just as suddenly, it would come back stronger than ever. People lived in almost constant fear. Can you imagine what the world would be like if this monster were still loose today?

The variola virus is the method by which smallpox spreads. A virus cannot be cured. However, the human immune system can fight it. A vaccine is an injection that prevents people from getting sick. It can be

Key Concepts

determined *adj.* serious and persistent
epidemic *n.* a disease that affects many people at the same time

made from a dead or weakened virus. The vaccine gives people a very weak case of the disease they need to be protected against. Once inside the body, the person's healthy cells develop defenses against that disease. If a person is later exposed to the disease, the body already has the tools to destroy it. In modern American society, most children receive several vaccines for common diseases before they are old enough to go to school.

Edward Jenner was a surgeon who developed a smallpox vaccine in the 1790s. At that time, doctors and surgeons practiced medicine very differently than they do today. People considered surgery physical **labor**. Jenner did not want to attend a university, but his training allowed him to study smallpox. It took him years, but eventually Jenner's **experiments** were successful. His vaccine could not get rid of the disease completely, but it did stop the virus from spreading.

Jenner's insight and determination prevented the deaths of many people. He also proved that humans are not helpless against disease, and that sometimes fear can inspire people to do **ingenious** things.

Key Concepts

labor *n.* work, employment

experiment *n.* a test to prove an idea or theory

ingenious *adj.* clever, inventive

The World's Smallpox Epidemics

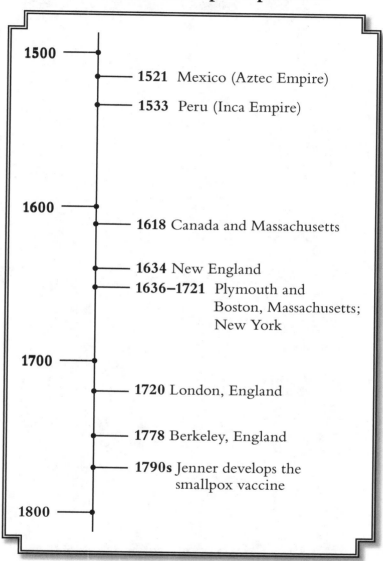

1500

1521 Mexico (Aztec Empire)

1533 Peru (Inca Empire)

1600

1618 Canada and Massachusetts

1634 New England

1636–1721 Plymouth and
Boston, Massachusetts;
New York

1700

1720 London, England

1778 Berkeley, England

1790s Jenner develops the
smallpox vaccine

1800

Visitors from Afar

*Spanish explorers brought disease
to the Aztec empire in Mexico.*

By 1521 the powerful Aztec empire of Mexico had had two visitors from far away. The first was Hernán Cortés, a tall, black-bearded Spanish adventurer with **hard, piercing** eyes and a voice that "echoed like thunder." Backed by fewer than six hundred Spanish soldiers and thousands of Indian allies who wanted freedom from Aztec domination, Cortés attacked their capital, Tenochtitlán. Built on the site of present-day Mexico City, it was home to some 225,000 people, making it several times larger than most European capitals at the time. Although the Spanish had guns and horses, the Aztecs had **superior numbers and by rights should have beaten them**.

That they failed to do so was **on account of** the second visitor to the Aztec empire—an invisible killer. Historians believe it arrived in the body of an African slave aboard a Spanish supply ship from Cuba. The invisible killer was a disease called smallpox.

....

hard, piercing intense

superior numbers and by rights should have beaten them
more soldiers and, therefore, should have defeated the
Spanish

on account of because of

Why Smallpox Killed the Aztecs But Few Spanish

Most of the Spanish soldiers with Cortés probably had had smallpox as children. Their bodies had developed what we today call **an immunity** to it, and so it could no longer make them sick. But the peoples of the Americas had never been exposed to smallpox. Both the Aztecs and Cortés's Indian allies had no resistance to it, and the result was disastrous.

Cortés's chaplain and biographer, Francisco Lopez de Gómara, described how the disease covered victims' bodies with vile sores, destroyed families, and **paralyzed** community life. "It spread from one Indian to another, and they, being so numerous and eating and sleeping together, quickly infected the whole country. In most houses all the occupants died, for, since it was their custom to bathe as a cure for all diseases, they bathed and were struck down." The Spaniard continues:

> *Those who did survive, having scratched themselves [raw], were left in such a condition that they frightened the others with the many deep pits on their faces, hands, and bodies. And then **came famine**, not because of want of bread, but of meal [to make it with], for the women do nothing but grind maize between two stones and bake it. The women, then, fell sick of the smallpox, bread failed, and many died of hunger. The corpses stank so horribly that no one would bury them; the streets were filled with them; and the officials, in order to **remedy** this situation, pulled the houses down to cover the corpses.*

....

an immunity a resistance; a defense
paralyzed completely stopped
came famine *they had no food*
remedy *stop*

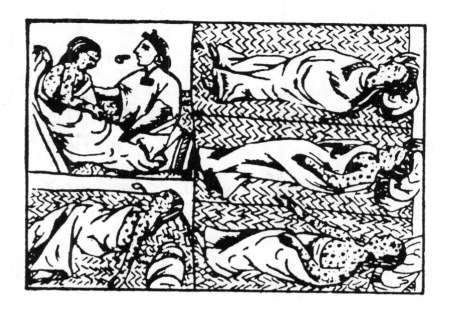

During the Spanish conquest of Mexico, a smallpox epidemic struck the Aztecs and the Indian allies of the Spanish in 1521. In these pictures—which were redrawn from illustrations by an eyewitness and first appeared in a book called the *Florentine Codex*—afflicted Aztecs hopelessly await the end.

PHOTO IN AUTHOR'S COLLECTION

Smallpox struck Cortés's allies, too. Yet that did not reduce his strength **in relation to** the Aztecs, since Indians died in the same **proportion** everywhere. His Spanish soldiers with their guns and horses remained intact, however. Of the few Spanish soldiers who died, nearly all **fell** in battle, not as smallpox victims.

Tragic as it was, the smallpox outbreak of 1521 was not the first, nor would it be the last, of its kind. It was but an incident in a far larger story that began long before the start of recorded history—the story of **infectious** diseases and how they attack people.

....

in relation to compared to
proportion large numbers
fell died
infectious contagious

BEFORE YOU MOVE ON...

1. **Text Features** How are the subheads on pages 13–14 different from the chapter title? How do they help you?

2. **Conclusions** Reread page 14. Why did smallpox affect the Aztecs and not the Spanish soldiers?

LOOK AHEAD Read pages 16–20 to find out where human diseases originally came from.

A Journey
to the Long-Ago Time

People were exposed to animal bacteria when they began to farm.

For **untold** generations, people lived not in tribes or nations, but in countless small family groups that wandered about, gathering wild plants and hunting animals to eat. About nine thousand years ago, however, humans began to change their way of living. Peoples in different parts of the world learned to grow plants like wheat, rice, and **maize** for food. Along with that, they began raising cattle, horses, sheep, goats, and pigs, turning wild animals into tame ones that would work for them.

These developments allowed the wanderers to settle down. With a larger food supply, their numbers increased steadily. Over time, scattered farms grew into villages, villages into towns and cities. Nations and empires **arose**. The first civilizations began in the broad river valleys of Asia and the Middle East. People invented writing and mathematics, studied the **heavens**, and devised the calendar to help them plant and harvest crops at the right time. All this was

....

untold many

maize corn

arose were formed

heavens stars and planets

real progress, but it came **at a hidden cost**. It exposed humanity to animal diseases.

All groups of living things, including humans, **are subject to** certain diseases that affect only that group. But sometimes a disease that affects one life-form may manage to "cross over" and infect an entirely different kind of life-form. During humanity's early history, animal diseases had little chance of infecting bands of wandering hunter-gatherers, who seldom camped in the same place for more than a few days at a time. Even if a disease did cross over to humans, the band was too small to keep it going. It might wipe out that particular group, but then the disease died out for lack of more people to infect. Deadly as it might be, it could not **gain a foothold elsewhere**.

That changed when large, permanent human settlements arose. Farmers lived close to their animals—close to their feces, urine, breath, blood, blisters, and sores. Often, to prevent theft, they kept prize animals in their homes. Farmers also collected animal wastes to use as crop fertilizer. Such close contact made it possible, over time, for the microbes that cause certain animal diseases to adapt to human "hosts"—a host is any living being, animal or plant, *on* which or *in* which another organism lives. According to historian William H. McNeill, "Most and probably all of the distinctive infectious diseases of civilization transferred to human populations from animal herds."

We are familiar with some of these diseases, though not **with their origins** in farm animals. For example, tuberculosis originated in cattle, influenza in pigs and ducks, and the common cold in horses. We share sixty-five diseases, including measles and whooping cough, with "man's best friend," the dog. Rats and mice, attracted by the farmers' stored

....

at a hidden cost with unexpected problems
are subject to can become sick from
gain a foothold elsewhere spread to others
with their origins from where they began

food, carry no fewer than thirty-two diseases to humans, including bubonic plague. Also known as the Black Death, that disease killed at least one in four Europeans between 1346 and 1352.

How Bacteria Can Cause Disease

Microscopic, single-celled organisms called bacteria cause many diseases. All life-forms—bacteria, plants, fungi, animals—consist of one or more cells. Whether it is the single cell of a bacterium or any of the 10 trillion cells that form an adult person, the cell is generally considered the smallest unit of life that we know. We say a cell is alive because it can take in and digest food, **excrete** waste, and thereby grow and reproduce. In more advanced life-forms, like people and animals, groups of cells work together with amazing harmony and coordination—some might even say intelligence—to form nerves, skin, bone, lungs, liver, and other organs and systems. The master plan for this intelligence is a large, information-packed molecule called DNA. Every cell (with a few exceptions) has DNA in its central core, or nucleus. DNA is a set of chemical instructions that cause the cell to make all the different things needed for its life and **specialized duties**.

Cells reproduce by making copies of themselves. In preparation for this, a cell first **increases production of** each of the thousands of different kinds of molecules within it, until it has doubled its contents. The DNA molecules within the cell are also copied, in a process called replication. When all is ready, the cell **elongates**, with half of the cell material going to one end and half to the other. In the final step,

....

excrete get rid of
specialized duties different responsibilities
increases production of makes many copies of
elongates becomes longer

called fission, this double-sized cell pinches off in the middle and separates into two daughter cells, each identical to the original one. These two cells can themselves divide; and so on. Not only simple bacterial cells but most of the cells in your body reproduce this way.

Bacteria live everywhere. Scientists have found them in clouds above mountaintops, in oil wells three miles deep, and near the mouths of undersea volcanoes. Bacteria live all over our skin, our hair, and even inside us. Nobody knows how many types of bacteria there are, only that the number is probably in the tens of thousands.

We do know that bacteria can enter our bodies through the air we breathe, breaks in our skin, spoiled food, polluted water, and sexual activity. Once inside, bacteria may cause disease by attacking certain cells, with the result that **vital organs** like the heart or lungs are damaged. Furthermore, bacteria can release poisons, called toxins, into our bodies that then circulate and cause **various kinds of cellular weakening and breakdown**. Yet most bacteria seem harmless to humans, and many are helpful to the way we live. Some bacteria feed on dead animals and plants, and thus keep the world from filling with garbage. Many living creatures make use of the basic chemicals— waste products—that are left over from this process. The bacteria in our intestines produce enzymes, chemicals that break down food into simpler materials. Though they do not "intend" to do so, these bacteria help us digest our food more completely.

Bacteria are life-forms visible only with the aid of a microscope. Yet they are giants in size compared to viruses, another major cause of disease. Thousands of viruses can fit inside a single bacterium. *Virus* comes from the Latin word meaning "a poisonous force."

Many scientists do not consider viruses true organisms—living

....

vital organs organs needed for survival

various kinds of cellular weakening and breakdown cells to become weak and die

beings—at all. They would say that viruses exist on the borderline of life. In terms of structure, a virus is less than a single cell—much less. It is really no more than a small amount of DNA. Viruses can be so small because they do not try to reproduce themselves on their own. Instead, they invade living cells and take advantage of all the elaborate structures and chemicals available there. By inserting a small amount of its own DNA into a cell's programming machinery, a virus forces the cell to **alter its operations**. Instead of putting its energy into growing and dividing, the cell is reprogrammed to manufacture more virus particles. In effect, the virus **hijacks** the cell's set of plans and installs its own. The new viruses—thousands of them—leave the host to invade nearby cells. Thus, viruses exist by killing or damaging host cells.

Life has **evolved** in such a way that different viruses have specialized in attacking specific plants or animals. Certain viruses attack human plant foods such as wheat, maize, sugarcane, soybeans, and potatoes. The animals we use for food are hosts to other kinds of viruses. Equally important, many human diseases are caused by viruses: colds, influenza, measles, mumps, chicken pox, polio, rabies, and AIDS, to name just a few. A virus also **unleashed** the Speckled Monster—smallpox—upon the Aztecs.

....

alter its operations change the way it does things
hijacks steals
evolved changed
unleashed started the spread of

BEFORE YOU MOVE ON...

1. **Cause and Effect** Reread pages 16–17. What happened when people began to settle in one place? How did this spread disease?

2. **Summarize** Reread pages 18–20. How do bacteria and viruses cause disease?

LOOK AHEAD Read pages 21–32 to find out what causes smallpox.

The *Biography* of a Killer Virus

Smallpox was first detected 8,000 years ago.

Scientists believe that smallpox is a fairly young disease. About eight thousand years ago, they think, the **ancestor of the** smallpox virus lived in an unknown farm animal somewhere in Asia or the Middle East. That virus probably made **its host animal** sick, but not sick enough to kill it. Then, in some way that is still unclear, the virus crossed over to a person. Perhaps the virus's DNA mutated, or changed, in a chance way that allowed this to happen. Whatever the case, the virus and **its descendants** survived in a person by attacking human cells. Because the victim either died or fought off the disease, the viruses did not attack every cell in the person's body.

The first smallpox victim whose name we have is the Egyptian ruler Ramses V, who died in 1157 B.C. His mummy bears the killer's **telltale marks**: a sheet of pimples extending from head to toe. Later, in another part of the world, Chinese doctors described smallpox in their writings. As the centuries passed, travelers spread the disease along the trade routes connecting Africa, Asia, and the Middle East.

....

ancestor of the original
its host animal the animal it was living in
its descendants other forms of it
telltale marks specific or unique symptom

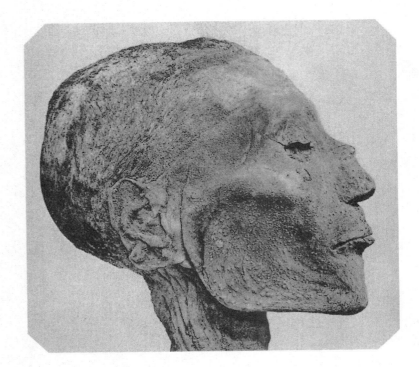

The oldest smallpox victim whose name we know. This mummified face of the ancient Egyptian ruler Ramses V still bears the telltale pockmarks after three thousand years.

Christian traders and crusaders then brought it back to Europe from **the Holy Land**.

Variola is the scientific name for the virus that causes smallpox. This word comes from *varius*—Latin for "spotted" or "speckled"—and is used to describe the masses of closely spaced red pimples that are a symptom of the disease. This is the symptom that gave rise to the term *Speckled Monster*. *Variola* got the name *smallpox* in the early 1500s, when syphilis, a **sexually transmitted disease native to the New World, began its march** across Europe. Since early-stage syphilis produces large pus blisters called pocks, English people called it the "great pox"—in contrast to variola, or the "small pox." The word *pox* refers to any rash consisting of pustules, or skin **lesions** filled with pus.

....

the Holy Land Israel

sexually transmitted disease native to the New World, began its march disease from America that spread by having sex, began to spread

lesions blisters, bubbles

How Smallpox Spreads

Variola belongs to a large group of viruses called the orthopoxviruses, or "true pox" viruses. Among its cousins are a **multitude** of diseases named after the creatures they infect. A partial list includes cowpox, swinepox, rabbitpox, camelpox, monkeypox, skunkpox, deerpox, buffalopox, sealpox, canarypox, turkeypox, gerbilpox, pigeonpox, crocodilepox, butterflypox, mothpox, mosquitopox, and grasshopperpox. All of these viruses carry genetic instructions—DNA—similar to variola. Yet none of these have **crossed over to** people—as far as we can tell. Chicken pox, however, is not caused by a poxvirus at all but by a member of the unrelated group of herpesviruses.

Nobody actually saw individual variola viruses until 1947. That year American scientists studied it with the powerful electron microscope. They found that variola is rectangular in shape, measuring $\frac{12}{1,000,000}$ (twelve one-millionths) of an inch in length. Three *million* variola would **scarcely** cover the period at the end of this sentence.

Scientists do not believe that variola has any animal carriers, so it cannot reproduce outside the human body. **A highly contagious disease**, it passes easily from person to person. Victims "leak" variola from sores in their throats and open blisters on their bodies. Each cough sprays up to five thousand invisible droplets of virus-filled saliva and mucus ten feet in every direction; a person who inhales even a few of these will most likely get infected. For example, when a smallpox victim was quarantined, or isolated, in a German hospital in 1970, seventeen patients became infected, some of

....

multitude large amount

crossed over to infected

scarcely barely; not even

A highly contagious disease A disease that spreads quickly

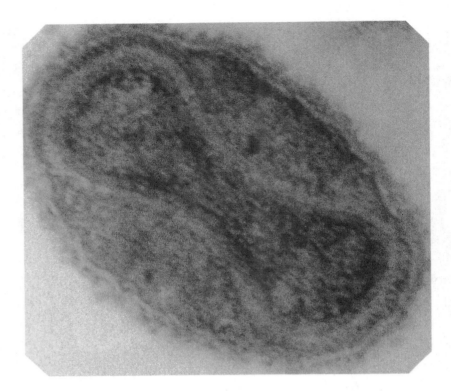

Portrait of a killer. This photograph of the variola virus, taken through an electron microscope, shows it enlarged millions of times. Among the largest of all viruses, variola is rectangular shaped, having an outer membrane and a core area shaped like a dumbbell. PHOTO IN AUTHOR'S COLLECTION

them three floors above his room. To find out why, investigators placed a smoke-generating machine in the patient's room. They discovered that air currents rising in a nearby stairwell had carried the virus to the upper floors.

Like all viruses, variola is a sneak thief. It begins its invasion **stealthily, without alerting its victim, until it has taken firm hold**. During the first ten days, its DNA takes over a few cells, usually in the throat. During that time, the victim feels fine. By day twelve, however, the virus has reproduced itself millions of times over. Huge numbers of viruses have left their host cells and are now traveling throughout the victim's body by way of the bloodstream.

....

stealthily, without alerting its victim, until it has taken firm hold quietly, without letting the victim know he or she is sick right away

The Symptoms of Smallpox

Early symptoms of smallpox are high fever, **splitting** headaches, muscle aches, violent stomach cramps, and vomiting. A rash appears on the roof of the mouth, face, hands, and arms. By day eighteen, the entire surface of the body is a mass of tiny red specks resembling a heat rash or flea bites. Gradually, these turn into pustules, blisters the size of peas, filled with a sticky yellowish white fluid called pus.

Around the year A.D. 350, a Chinese doctor named Ho Kung accurately described the onset of smallpox. "Recently," he wrote, "there have been persons suffering from epidemic sores which attack the head, face, and trunk. In a short time, these sores spread all over the body. They have the appearance of hard **boils**, containing white matter. While some of the pustules are drying up, a fresh crop appears."

Life becomes **a torment**. Every inch of the victim's skin feels as if it is on fire. Pus glues swollen eyelids together. The body **gives off a nauseating odor**. If the virus attacks a vital organ—heart, lungs, liver, kidneys, brain—death comes by day thirty at the latest. If not, scabs the size of a pencil eraser form over the pustules and fall off a few weeks later.

The Speckled Monster generally killed one out of every three of its victims. Survivors bore its marks for the rest of their lives. One in six went blind in one or both eyes. In everyone, the disease left small, deep scars, called pockmarks. Each pockmark was like a pit scooped out of the skin. Yet, in a way, these survivors were the lucky ones, whatever their suffering might have been. For the disease would never trouble them again, thanks to the human body's natural defense against disease—the amazing immune system.

....

splitting very painful

boils pimples

a torment horrible; like torture

gives off a nauseating odor smells horrible

How Our Bodies Fight Disease

The main purpose of our powerful and complex immune system is to recognize invading microbes—organisms of microscopic size—and destroy them. Because bacteria and viruses come in almost unimaginable and ever-changing variety, our immune system cannot know in advance what an invader will look like. What it *can* do is **patrol** the inside of our bodies, looking for what is not normally present.

The job of recognizing foreign invaders is carried out by a special **class** of immune cells called lymphocytes, which circulate through our blood and lymphatic vessels. One kind, the "B" lymphocytes, or B cells, carry molecules on their surface called antibodies. Antibodies are designed to stick to other molecules, and they are made in such a tremendous variety of shapes that at least one is usually able to stick to any new invading microbe—for instance, to a molecule present on the surface of an invading bacterial cell. (Any molecule to which an antibody sticks is called an antigen.) Then the B cell goes into action. Over the next fourteen days, it divides again and again until a huge number of B cells with those particular antibodies have **accumulated**. During the fourteen-day period, the B cells sometimes make small changes to their antibodies so that they will stick even more tightly to the **antigen** on the invader.

Then other cells of the immune system, large white blood cells called phagocytes ("cell eaters"), come in to destroy the antibody-coated bacteria. To guard against future infections by the same kind of bacteria, a percentage of the B cells that stick to those particular bacteria are kept available even after the infection has

....

patrol search throughout
class group
accumulated gathered
antigen disease-fighting substance

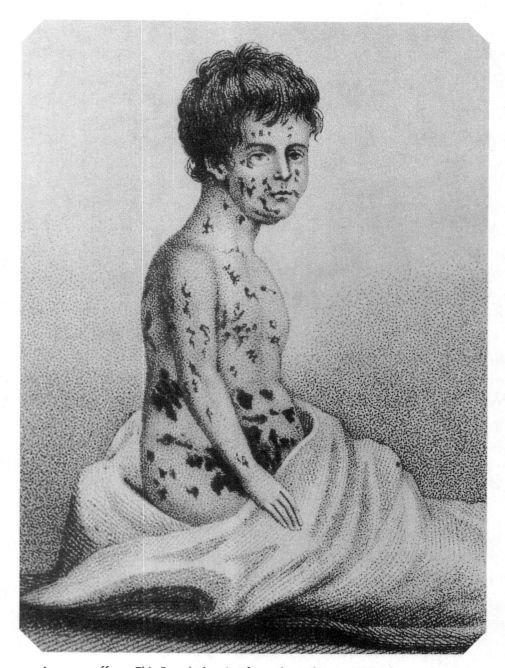

A young sufferer. This French drawing from about the year 1830 shows a boy covered with smallpox pustules, some of which are so close together that they seem to form large skin blotches. PHOTO COURTESY OF THE NATIONAL LIBRARY OF MEDICINE

been beaten. These "memory B cells" remain in the body for years, even for a lifetime, and allow the immune system to respond much more quickly—in two or three days instead of fourteen—if the same kind of bacteria attempt to invade again. Having such memory cells in our **circulation** gives us *immunity*, so that we can quickly fight off future infections—often so quickly and efficiently that we aren't even aware it is happening.

B cells are some help in fighting virus infections, too, by recognizing viruses traveling through the bloodstream and targeting them for destruction. But they cannot help when a virus has already **gained entrance to** the inside of a cell. To solve this problem, the immune system has a second kind of lymphocyte, called T cells, which also patrol our bodies looking for things that shouldn't be there. Instead of antibodies, T cells carry another kind of sticky molecule on their surface. T cells can sense whether a cell is normal or has been invaded by a virus, because virus-infected cells display telltale molecules on their surface. Once a T cell has identified an infected cell, it calls in specialized killer cells to destroy it. At the final cleanup stage, once again the large white blood cells called phagocytes approach the infected cells, break them apart, and digest them. Pus consists in part of the **liquefied remains** of phagocytes that have died after killing infected cells, as well as other cell waste products.

During this whole process, the body may produce a high fever, which is one reason why you feel sick before you begin to feel well. Some researchers believe a high fever is one of the body's way of limiting a virus's ability to take over cells.

As with B cells, after a virus infection has been **fought off** there are also "memory T cells" that remain in our blood so that the

....

circulation blood
gained entrance to entered
liquefied remains liquid waste
fought off destroyed

immune system can respond quickly and strongly to any future infections by the same virus or a very similar one. Immunity may last for several years or for life, depending on the invader. Smallpox survivors have lifetime immunity.

The Effects of Smallpox on Its Victims

Until about two centuries ago, English people used to say, "From smallpox and love few remain free." It was true. People everywhere saw a visit from the Speckled Monster as a normal, if dreadful, part of growing up. When it struck a community, it killed everyone whose immune system could not **cope with the assault**; for example, **poorly nourished people** are less able to fight off a disease than the well nourished. Yet as the number of survivors grew, the virus seemed to fade away for lack of anyone unexposed to receive it.

Years later, however, it would return to a population, brought by outsiders. Most adults were already immune, having had it as children or teenagers. But not the new **crop** of children! Everyone born since the last outbreak was human "fuel" for the raging virus. Many died. As before, those who managed to survive never got it again, and the disease seemed to fade away—until next time. This explains another **folk** saying: "No man dares count his children as his own until after they have had the smallpox."

Smallpox forced families to make frightful choices. Seeing a loved one shrieking in pain, becoming a swollen mass of oozing pustules, tore at family members' hearts. Yet keeping the sick at home might destroy an entire family. Dr. William Buchan discussed the dilemma in his book, *Domestic Medicine*, printed in 1769.

....

cope with the assault fight it

poorly nourished people people who do not eat well

crop generation, group

folk common

*If an infant happen to be **seized with** the smallpox upon the mother's breast, who has not had the disease herself, the scene must be distressing. If she **continue to suckle the child it is at the peril of her own life; if she wean it in all probability it will perish**. How often is the affectionate mother forced to leave her house and abandon her children at the very time when her care is most necessary? Yet should parental affection get the better of her fears the consequences would often prove fatal.*

Many ignored the danger and nursed the victim as best they could. Many others did just the opposite. At about the same time that Dr. Buchan wrote his book, another English doctor noted how "the husband forsakes the wife, the mother her children, and the son his father." Terrified, family members either ran away or put the sufferer out of the house, to die alone in the woods or by the roadside.

The Speckled Monster also shaped people's ideas of female beauty. An English nobleman, Sir Henry Sidney, and his wife, Mary, learned this in the 1580s. When called away on urgent business, Sir Henry had to leave his wife behind. He came home a few weeks later, only to find her changed. "I left her a full fair lady," he wrote sadly, "and when I returned I found her as foul a lady as the smallpox could make her." Hating herself, Lady Mary broke all her mirrors and spent the rest of her life alone in a darkened room. In old Europe, smallpox scarred so many women's faces that anyone with an unmarked face was considered beautiful.

Nobody knew what caused smallpox. People blamed it on God's anger, poisonous gases seeping from the earth, and "imbalances" in victims' body fluids. Lacking a true understanding of the disease, any "treatment," however bizarre, seemed better than just standing

....

seized with *infected by*

continue to suckle the child it is at the peril of her own life; if she wean it in all probability it will perish *continues to breast-feed her child, she risks her life; if she does not feed her child, it will probably die*

30

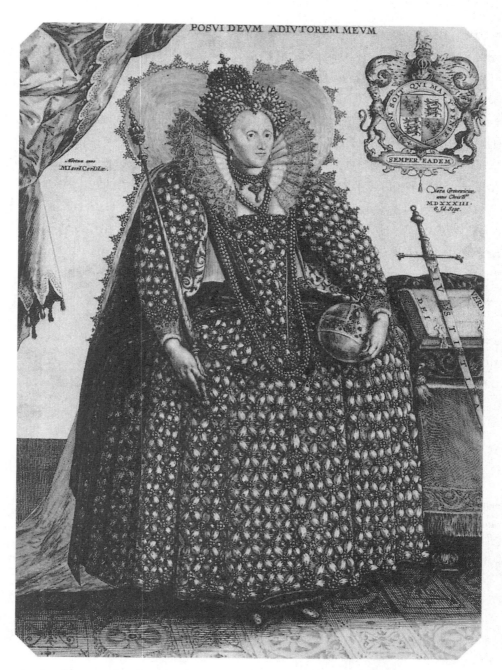

Smallpox struck rich and poor, noble and commoner, with equal ferocity. Although she survived an attack in the mid-1500s, the disease left Queen Elizabeth I of England nearly bald and without eyebrows.

by and watching people suffer. Doctors gave patients powerful emetics—drugs to make them vomit—or had them drink "tonics" of powdered horse manure, mouse whiskers, lye soap, and chopped sponge, to fight the disease. Holding a rag soaked in vinegar over your nose, or carrying a bag of **camphor** around your neck, was also supposed to **ward off** infection.

Doctors used heat to **"draw out"** the fever. Thus, they wrapped patients in woolen blankets and made them lie beside a roaring fire even in summertime. Similarly, doctors used the "red treatment" to draw out the fever. Since they considered red a "warm" color, they hung red curtains around patients' beds, put red caps on their heads, and had them drink the juice of red berries. When Queen Elizabeth I of England got smallpox in 1562, at the age of twenty-nine, the royal doctors wrapped her in a heavy red blanket and put her close to a fireplace filled with huge burning logs. She survived and lived to the age of seventy, but the disease left her nearly bald, without eyebrows, and her face pitted with deep scars. For the rest of her life, Elizabeth I wore a red wig and heavy makeup on her face. At best, such treatments as she suffered did not affect the disease at all. At worst, they killed the patient before the disease **ran its course**.

....

camphor medicine
ward off prevent
"draw out" reduce; bring down
ran its course killed the person

BEFORE YOU MOVE ON...

1. **Sequence** Reread pages 23–24. What happens when the variola virus infects a person?

2. **Viewing** Look at the drawing and caption on page 27. How does it help you understand smallpox better?

LOOK AHEAD Read pages 33–45 to learn how smallpox changed North America.

The Speckled Monster Helps Conquer the New World

European explorers spread smallpox around the world.

Smallpox was more even than a personal or a social tragedy. The disease is so **lethal** and contagious that it shaped the history of the New World **down to** the present. Until Christopher Columbus's voyage of 1492, the **vastness** of the "Ocean Sea" (the Atlantic Ocean) had kept the New World isolated from the rest of the world—and its diseases. Native people, who had never been exposed to smallpox, had no immunity to it. That gave the Spanish and, later, other European invaders a huge advantage in the struggles that followed.

The Speckled Monster, traveling with the Spanish, killed more native peoples than anything else. The Aztecs, said an unnamed soldier, "die so easily that the bare look and smell of a Spaniard causes them to **give up the ghost**." Variola, not Spanish guns or brains or courage, conquered the Aztecs. Just how many died is unclear. Historians believe smallpox killed half the Aztecs within six months. Worse, in less than a century the total native population of Mexico, including the Aztecs, fell from about 25 million to just over a million,

---

lethal deadly

down to until

vastness great size

give up the ghost die

largely due to this disease.

In 1533 smallpox allowed another Spaniard, Francisco Pizarro, to overthrow the Inca empire in Peru. The Inca, an ingenious people who built stone-paved roads better than any found in Europe, were helpless against the invisible enemy. Variola killed their ruler and as many as 250,000 of his **subjects**. And that was just the first outbreak! After that, no year passed without variola **rearing its ugly head** somewhere in Peru. "They died by scores and hundreds," a Spanish priest reported in 1585. "**Villages were depopulated.** Corpses were scattered over the fields or piled up in the houses or huts."

French explorers brought the Speckled Monster to the tribes of eastern Canada. In 1618 a Catholic missionary, Father Le Jeune, wrote of "the great epidemic which has slain nearly all these peoples, without getting any hold of the French." About the same time, the disease tore through Native American villages along the Massachusetts coast. We do not know where it came from; there were no white settlements near the worst-hit areas. Perhaps sailors brought it when they came ashore for fresh water. What is certain is that it killed nine out of ten coastal Indians. Unable to cope with this horror, the survivors abandoned their villages and fled to neighbors, taking the virus with them.

The early history of the English colonies in North America is also the history of smallpox. In 1634, for example, the Wampanoag, a tribe living near Plymouth Colony, quarreled with the newcomers over land. Then, the English said, God favored them with a "miracle." The Almighty sent "the pox" to the "heathen savages."

That pleased Governor William Bradford. "Whole towns of them were swept away," he wrote in his book *Of Plymouth Plantation: 1620–1647*. "They die like rotten sheep [and are] not able to help

....

subjects people

rearing its ugly head reappearing

Villages were depopulated. Many people died in the villages.

one another; no, not to make a fire, nor to fetch a little water to drink, nor to bury the dead. But by the marvelous goodness of God not one of the English was so much as sick." Today, we would **condemn such a remark for its ferocious inhumanity**, its dividing the world into good people (English) and evil ones (Indians). Yet Bradford did not see things as we do. A deeply religious Puritan, he believed Bible history was being repeated in the New World. God had once helped the Israelites conquer the Holy Land and slay its "heathen" inhabitants. Now, Bradford believed, He sent smallpox to rid New England of "red heathens" so "Godly people," the Puritans, could settle the country.

Bradford spoke too soon. The Speckled Monster had not forgotten the settlers. Although many had survived the disease and become immune to it before leaving Europe, many others, especially children, had yet to catch it. Between 1636 and 1721, smallpox struck Plymouth, Boston, New York, and other **colonial** towns four times. **But all was not lost.** For by the early 1700s, people were learning how to defend themselves against this horrible visitor.

....

condemn such a remark for its ferocious inhumanity
criticize a person who said such bad things

colonial newly settled

But all was not lost. But there was hope.

$\mathcal{F}$ighting Back with Inoculation

Inoculation became popular in Europe.

$\mathcal{A}$bout the year A.D. 950, by the Western calendar, an unknown man or woman in China made an important discovery. We cannot say *how* the discovery happened, only that it did. This person probably noticed that people who got smallpox and survived never seemed to get the disease a second time. It did not matter whether, during their illness, they had only a few scabs or were completely covered by them. If they lived, they never developed the symptoms of smallpox again. Why? **Presumably** no one back then knew what we now know about the human immune system and how it works. Even so, the protective effects of the immune system were clear enough.

That person, whoever he or she was, tried something quite remarkable. She, let's say, peeled the scabs off a recovering smallpox patient and ground them into a fine powder. Taking a hollow reed, she then blew the powder up the noses of healthy people who had never had the disease. This is called insufflation.

If we try to imagine **the reasoning behind her curious behavior**, one explanation stands out. She must have figured out the scabs were connected to getting the disease—and giving it. Her idea

....

Presumably It is likely that

the reasoning behind her curious behavior what she was thinking

36

was probably to give people a mild case of smallpox—hoping to spare them from **a full-blown attack**—so that they would survive and be free of the disease for the rest of their lives. We do not know how much scab powder she used, but her system worked. For about a week, patients ran a fever, developed small pustules and scabs—and then recovered. After that, the Speckled Monster seemed to pass them by.

Today, an immunologist might explain this by saying that the immune system of the donor, the person who "donated" the scabs, had already weakened or killed the viruses in the scabs. When introduced into another person as a powder, they **triggered** the B cells of that person's immune system to produce antibodies. Then the T cells got involved, and the rest of the immune system, finally **leading to lasting immunity to** future infections.

Knowledge of Inoculation Spreads

Traders spread the Chinese practice across Asia. By the late 1600s, it had reached westward all the way to the Turkish empire. By then, however, things were being done differently. Instead of blowing scab powder up a healthy person's nose, a drop or two of pus was taken from a person with a mild case of smallpox and rubbed into a scratch made with a needle in someone else's upper arm. Today, we call this practice inoculation. The word comes from *in oculare*, Latin for "giving eyes"—a term for an ancient gardening trick. Gardeners would attach "eyes," or buds, from a prized plant to another plant through cuts in the stem. This grafting made the plant healthier and gave it tastier fruit.

....

a full-blown attack becoming very sick

triggered caused

leading to lasting immunity to preventing the person from ever getting

Europeans knew little about Turkey, and less about inoculation. That began to change, thanks to two Greek doctors, Emanuel Timoni and Giacomo Pylarini, who had visited the Turkish capital, Constantinople (now called Istanbul). In 1713, Dr. Timoni sent a report on inoculation to the Royal Society of London, **an organization devoted to spreading** useful knowledge. Dr. Pylarini issued a small book on inoculation two years later. These writings became known only to a tiny group of learned people, however. To capture the public's attention, inoculation needed "social clout," a push from people of high rank in society. We would call them celebrities.

That push came from a brave woman, Lady Mary Wortley Montagu, the wife of Britain's ambassador to Turkey. Once a great beauty, Lady Mary knew the Speckled Monster all too well. Smallpox had left her with a scarred face and no eyelashes; it had also killed her younger brother. Calling herself Flavia, after an ancient Roman woman, she described her feelings about her lost beauty in a poem:

> *The wretched Flavia on her couch reclined;*
> *Thus breathed the anguish of a wounded mind,*
> *A glass [mirror] reversed in her tight hand she bore,*
> *For now she **shunned the face she sought before**.*
> *'How am I changed! alas! how am I grown*
> *A frightful **spectre** to myself unknown!*
> *Where's my complexion? where city radiant bloom,*
> *That promised happiness for years to come? . . .*
> *No art can give me back my beauty lost.*
> *In tears, surrounded by my friends, I lay*
> *Masked o'er, and trembled at the sight of day; . . .*

....

an organization devoted to spreading a group of people who worked to spread

shunned the face she sought before *looked away from the face she once liked*

spectre *ghost*

> . . . [L]et me live in some deserted place,
> There hide in shades this lost inglorious face.'

Yet Lady Mary did not hide in the shadows. She did not let those pockmarks destroy her self-confidence. A likable person, she made friends easily, traveled widely, and took an interest in everything.

In April 1717, she described inoculation in a letter to her friend Sarah Chiswell:

> I am going to tell you a thing that will make you wish yourself here. The smallpox, **so fatal and so general** among us, is here entirely harmless. . . . There is a set of old women, who make it their business to perform the operation. . . . [Turkish] people . . . make parties for this purpose, and when they are met (commonly fifteen or sixteen together) the old woman comes with a nutshell full of the matter of the best type of smallpox, and asks what vein you please to have opened. She immediately rips open **that** you offer her, with a large needle . . . and puts into the vein as much **matter** as can lie on the head of her needle, and after that, binds up the little wound. . . . Every year, thousands undergo this operation. . . . I am well satisfied with the safety of the experiment, since I intend to try it on my dear little son.

True to her word, Lady Mary secretly had her six-year-old son, Edward, inoculated. A week later she told her husband about it; the child had recovered fully.

The Montagu family returned to England in 1720. Early the next year, smallpox struck London, the nation's capital and the largest city in the world. It raced through the population, killing hundreds each

----

so fatal and so general *so deadly and common*
that *the vein*
matter *of the smallpox*
True to her word Like she said she would

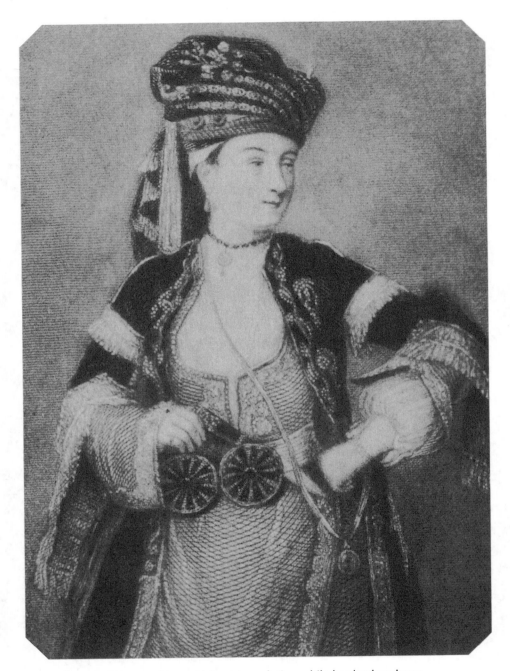

Lady Mary Montagu learned about inoculation while her husband was ambassador to Turkey in the early 1700s. She persuaded the royal family to introduce the practice to England. PHOTO COURTESY OF THE NATIONAL LIBRARY OF MEDICINE

week, including many children. To protect her three-year-old daughter, also named Mary, Lady Mary had a doctor inoculate her. As she expected, the child recovered without any ill effects. Newspapers picked up the story. Before long, inoculation was the talk of the city.

Lady Mary became a **champion** of inoculation. She thought everybody should be inoculated, and never missed a chance to say so. One day, Princess Caroline, wife of the future king, George II, invited her to the royal palace. Her Highness had two small daughters of her own and feared for their safety. She listened intently as her guest described the wonders of inoculation. It seemed too good to be true. So, before risking the young princesses' lives on a method as yet untried in England, she had the royal doctors test its safety.

Europe Tests the Inoculation

Test it how? Better yet, test it on whom? Surely not on persons of "quality"; that is, members of **the nobility**. In eighteenth-century Europe, nobles saw themselves as a special breed, **superior to** other humans. Their lives, they felt, were more valuable than those of simple "commoners." With that in mind, the royal doctors set out to find "unimportant" people, those nobody but their loved ones would miss if the test should fail and those inoculated die from smallpox.

In that summer of 1721, they visited Newgate, a London jail that held criminals awaiting execution. The English **were very free with** the death penalty. People as young as nine were hung not only for murder but also for burglary, stealing a silk handkerchief, and for hundreds of other, nonviolent crimes. The doctors found six prisoners—three men and three women—who had never had

....

champion supporter
the nobility royalty; rich and important people
superior to far better than
were very free with often used

smallpox. These six were offered something they could not refuse. Death by hanging was certain to come, and very soon. Of course, if they agreed to have the inoculation test and it failed, they would die, too. But if they survived their smallpox inoculation, they would be set free and, hopefully, never have to fear smallpox. All took the offer and survived.

After that, the doctors forced one of the prisoners, a young woman named Elizabeth Harrison, to take care of a ten-year-old girl with a raging case of smallpox. Every night for six weeks, Elizabeth had to sleep with the girl. The poor child coughed, spraying variola onto the sheets and pillows and into her bedmate's face. Yet Elizabeth did not get sick. That was a good sign indeed, but Princess Caroline demanded still further proof.

To be doubly sure of inoculation's safety, she ordered a test on children in a London orphanage. Nobody asked the orphans' **consent**. The doctors simply selected eleven boys and girls and inoculated them. All eleven did well. Convinced at last, Her Highness had her daughters inoculated at once. They recovered, too. After that, the royal family gave its blessing to inoculation. Many of England's "best people" rushed to get inoculated, to keep up with the latest royal fashion.

Despite these early successes, inoculation had enemies. Some **devout** Christians resisted efforts at preventing any disease. Diseases, they argued, did not have natural causes but came straight from heaven. They were "bolts of divine lightning," sent by God to punish sinners and warn others to **stay on the right path**. Thus, trying to prevent disease was wrong **on two counts**. It interfered with God's

....

consent permission
devout very religious
stay on the right path behave well
on two counts for two reasons

justice and it encouraged sinners in their evil ways. A London preacher, the Reverend Edmund Massey, put it this way: "The fear of disease **is a happy restraint to men**. . . . If men were more healthy, 'tis a great chance they would be less righteous."

Others objected to inoculation for health, rather than religious, reasons. Here the critics had a point. Over time, it turned out that inoculation was not as safe as Lady Mary and Princess Caroline's doctors supposed. From 1721 to 1732, records show, 474 people were inoculated in England. Of these, nine got smallpox and died; that is one in fifty. Why?

The trouble lay both with the doctors who performed the inoculations and the materials they used. Since doctors back then knew nothing about the immune system, good results owed more to luck than science. Sometimes, a doctor took pus before a donor's immune system had killed or weakened all the viruses sufficiently to use for inoculation; some Chinese doctors may also have peeled scabs off smallpox sufferers too soon. Moreover, inoculated persons **shed** millions of virus particles every time they coughed, sneezed, or exhaled. Dried pus and scabs shed from their bodies **contaminated** blankets and bed **linens**. So, although inoculation might protect one person, that person might give the disease to others who had not received an inoculation, chiefly members of their own families.

Despite the dangers, inoculation spread. Although risky, it was safer than an unplanned visit from the Speckled Monster. Sooner or later, nearly everybody would have **a bout** with smallpox. At least inoculation seemed a way to get a milder case of it, with less chance of dying. By the 1740s, it had become a business. European doctors got

....

is a happy restraint to men stops people from doing wrong

shed released, spread

contaminated infected, polluted

linens sheets

a bout an experience

rich by inoculating the wealthy. Dr. Thomas Dimsdale, of London, served Catherine the Great, empress of Russia. In return, Her Majesty made him a nobleman and gave him a treasure of gold, silver, and jewels. His countrymen Robert and Daniel Sutton, a father and son, inoculated over 2,500 people in five years. The Suttons charged £25 per inoculation, or about $3,000 in today's money.

How People Were Inoculated in the 1700s

Getting an inoculation was called "buying the pox." To prepare for the "purchase," patients had to go through a strict routine, itself almost a form of torture. A man described the ordeal of a boy he knew in 1760. "He was a fine, ruddy boy, and, at eight years of age was, with many others, put under a preparatory process for inoculation with the smallpox. This preparation lasted six weeks. He was bled to **ascertain** whether his blood was fine; was purged repeatedly, till he became **emaciated and feeble**; he was kept on a low diet . . . and dosed with a diet-drink to sweeten his blood." Bleeding involved a doctor making **an incision** in an arm vein and taking an ounce or two of blood. Purging meant "cleansing" the bowels with laxatives and enemas. Most patients were also made to vomit once a day; vomiting was brought on by drugs called emetics.

Since it was known that newly inoculated patients might spread the disease while they had it, they had to be isolated. Those who could afford the expense prepared for it in their own rooms, at home, cared for by servants who had already had smallpox. During that dangerous time, their families moved in with relatives. All others went to the "inoculation stables," large sheds built in the country or on the

....

ascertain find out; discover

emaciated and feeble thin and weak

an incision a cut

outskirts of towns. *Stables* was the right word for these awful places. Each held from twelve to fifteen people of different ages. Children and adults were treated alike. Everyone lay on a straw-filled mattress placed not on a bed but on the dirty floor. Those who had recently bought the pox were feverish. Crying children called for their parents. They ate twice a day—dry toast and weak tea.

Inoculated patients left the stables when their symptoms passed. Some went home too early, taking the virus with them and infecting others. Meanwhile, smallpox continued to kill the uninoculated majority in **droves**. During the eighteenth century, it **snuffed out the lives of** 400,000 people each year in Europe alone, out of a population of about 70 million.

Where would it end? Clearly, people needed a safer, cheaper, and more reliable way of **combating** the Speckled Monster. An English country doctor, Edward Jenner, found that way. His achievement has **placed him in the first rank of** heroes of science. If not for him, countless people living today would have died miserably or never have been born.

....

droves large numbers

snuffed out the lives of killed

combating fighting, treating

placed him in the first rank of made him one of the top

BEFORE YOU MOVE ON...

1. **Cause and Effect** Reread pages 33–35. What happened to the people of North America when European invaders brought smallpox?

2. **Problem and Solution** Reread pages 36–37. What were two ways to inoculate people before Dr. Jenner's time?

LOOK AHEAD Read pages 46–57 to find out how people in the 1700s felt about surgeons.

The Jenners of Berkeley

A young Jenner was influenced by a changing world.

Edward Jenner was born May 17, 1749, at Berkeley, a village in the farm country of western England. He came into the world in a time of great change. During his childhood, the chief European nations fought a series of bloody wars over territory, trading rights, and their colonies. Those violent years **also coincided with** the Age of Reason, a popular term for the eighteenth century, a time when people increasingly used **logic and scientific inquiry** to challenge comfortable traditions and superstitious beliefs. The Age of Reason influenced America, too. For example, in 1752, when Edward Jenner was three, Benjamin Franklin tied a key to a kite and flew it during a thunderstorm to prove his theory that lightning is electricity. When struck, a blue flash—electricity—shot out of the end of the key. Franklin used the knowledge he gained to invent the lightning rod, a piece of metal placed high on a building or ship to **conduct** lightning harmlessly into the ground or water.

Edward was the eighth of the nine children of the Reverend Stephen Jenner and his wife, Sarah. His parents were always busy, his father with his church duties and his mother with her chores. Soon

....

also coincided with occurred at the same time as

logic and scientific inquiry judgment and scientific questioning

conduct direct

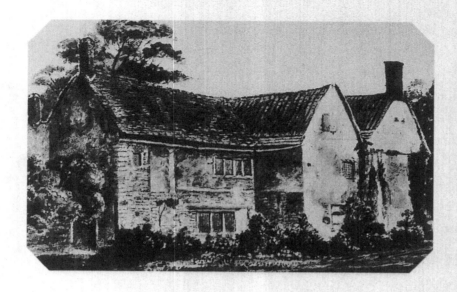

after Edward turned five, they died within a few weeks of each other. Eventually, the boy's elder brother, Stephen, also a minister, **took charge of** both him and their father's church.

We know very little about Edward Jenner's early years. He left no diaries, and his letters deal mostly with his medical practice, not **private matters**. Nor do we have any **portraits** of him as a youth, or descriptions of him by relatives or neighbors. As a child, he must have had playmates, but we have no record of their names. If he was like other country children, he would have fished in nearby streams, walked in the woods, and played games. Eighteenth-century English children **went in for** hide-and-seek, blindman's bluff, and a type of handball called fives.

Edward's brother, Stephen, seems to have been a gentle, loving person. At night, by candlelight, Stephen probably taught Edward how to read, write, and do sums—arithmetic. Many children at that time learned the basics from family members at home. When Edward

---

took charge of cared for
private matters his personal life
portraits pictures
went in for played games like

turned seven, Stephen enrolled him in a local private school. There he studied Greek and Latin, subjects he must master if he hoped to go to a university, as Stephen and their father had done. Although the Jenners had never been poor, they had never been rich, either. For Edward's education, that did not matter, since universities offered **generous scholarships** to the sons of **clergymen**. Yet Edward was **no scholar**, learning just enough to get by without a whipping for laziness. University study was not for him. So when Edward turned fourteen in 1763, Stephen sent him to live with Daniel Ludlow, a surgeon in the neighboring village of Chipping Sodbury, to learn his trade.

Being a Surgeon in the 1700s

Today surgeons are highly trained doctors of medicine. But that was not true in Jenner's day. In the 1700s in England, only those who had studied medicine at the universities of Oxford and Cambridge could use the title of doctor. A committee of doctors would give each graduate a test. If he passed, he was granted a license to practice medicine. Notice *he,* not *she.* Medicine was a profession open only to men. Women could not become doctors anywhere in Europe or America until the late 1800s.

Surgeons did not begin as doctors but as barber-surgeons. Barbers are handy with razors. They have to be, in order to shave people and cut their hair and beards and so on. Centuries before Jenner's birth, barbers began to make extra money by cutting open boils—infected areas on people's skin—and bleeding the sick. In time, some barbers gave up giving shaves and cutting hair in order to practice surgery full-time.

....

generous scholarships large amounts of money for school

clergymen men who worked in the church

no scholar not a very good student

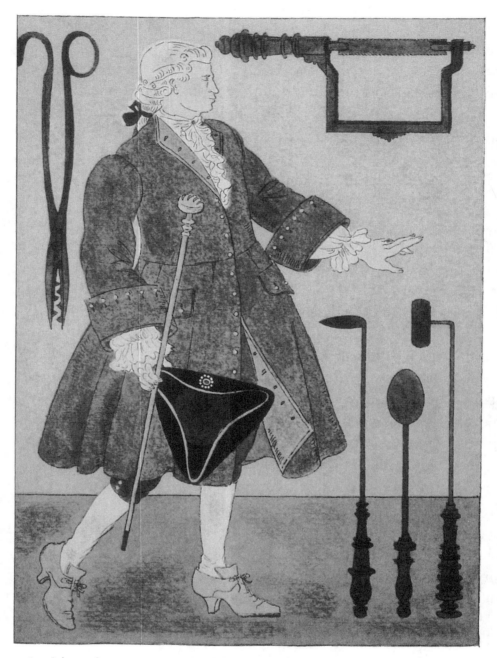

An eighteenth-century surgeon with his tools: saw, forceps, and various types of probes. In Edward Jenner's day, surgeons were not medical doctors, because they did not have university degrees. PHOTO COURTESY OF THE NATIONAL LIBRARY OF MEDICINE

Although surgeons performed operations, because they had no university education or medical licenses they lacked the respect given to doctors. Surgeons worked with blades. Back then, people thought of blades in the same way they thought of hammers and saws, pliers and plows—as tools of craftspeople, of **manual laborers**. In old Europe, only the lower classes earned a living with their hands. A "gentleman" did not soil his hands with physical labor. Such work was considered beneath his dignity. As an educated person, a doctor was a gentleman. He seldom touched a patient during an examination. Instead, he observed the patient, asked about symptoms, and looked at a urine sample; the urine's color and smell could offer clues to the patient's illness. Finally, the doctor chose a treatment, usually a drug, or **concoction**, of some kind. An apothecary, or druggist, prepared the medicine from various herbs and chemicals.

Although Jenner left no written account of his training, it probably was not much different from any other surgeon's. A young man learned surgery by living with an experienced surgeon, reading his medical books, and watching what he did. The **apprentice** did not take any tests, since only those who had attended a university were tested, and they had to know Latin well. Mostly, a young man learned surgery "by touch," as they said; that is, working as a surgeon's assistant. Surgeons called themselves Mister, never Doctor. Nor did they charge the same fees as doctors.

Each day, rain or shine, Jenner followed his master **on his rounds**. They rode on horseback, returning home long after dark. Like many surgeons, Mr. Ludlow was his own apothecary. At every stop, he gave out medicines he had prepared himself or with his assistant's help.

....

manual laborers people who worked with their hands

concoction mixture of ingredients

apprentice assistant

on his rounds as he visited patients

When necessary, he lanced boils, set broken bones, sewed up cuts, and pulled teeth. Farm accidents were common, so he **amputated** infected fingers, arms, and legs to prevent blood poisoning. Since there were no anesthetics—painkillers—he had to work quickly. As Mr. Ludlow would cut, Jenner would use all his strength to hold the patient down; husky farmhands were recruited to help, too.

Jenner turned twenty-one in 1770. By then, he seems to have learned all Mr. Ludlow had to teach him. Most young men his age would have been glad to **hang out their surgeon's shingle and start on their own**. Not Edward Jenner. He loved his work and wanted to be the best surgeon possible. Mr. Ludlow understood and arranged for him to study with a London surgeon, John Hunter. Brother Stephen agreed to pay all expenses. It proved to be a **worthy investment**.

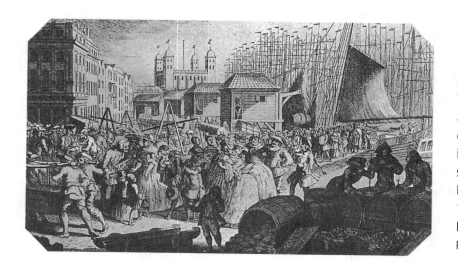

This 1757 view of London shows the waterfront along the Thames River. The largest city on earth at that time, London was overcrowded and dirty, ideal conditions for the spread of disease. From Louis Philippe Boitard, "The Imports of Great Britain from France."
PHOTO IN AUTHOR'S COLLECTION

....

amputated cut off; removed

hang out their surgeon's shingle and start on their own
leave Mr. Ludlow's practice and start their own

worthy investment good choice

The Young Surgeon

*A young Jenner learned
how to be a surgeon.*

A brilliant surgeon, John Hunter had **retired from** the British
army and now regularly took two or three students into his London
home. Soon after Jenner arrived, Hunter published his *Natural History
of the Human Teeth*, **a pioneering book in** dentistry, and began
work on a book about the treatment of gunshot wounds. Mr. Hunter
also had a huge collection of animal specimens and human organs
preserved in alcohol, which he kept in a private museum next to
his house. **Its prize specimen** was the complete skeleton of a man
named Charles O'Brien, over seven feet tall and known as "The
Irish Giant." Hunter had paid O'Brien for his skeleton years before
O'Brien died. You can still see it in the Hunterian Museum of the
Royal College of Surgeons, London, which is named in honor of
the great surgeon.

Mr. Hunter had a **ferocious** temper and, friends said, often let
loose with "the bitterest swearing." Nevertheless, he and his newest
pupil saw things in each other that they immediately liked. They
became lifelong friends. Dr. John Baron, another friend of Jenner's,
says in his *Life of Edward Jenner:* "The pupil not only respected the

....

retired from stopped working for

a pioneering book in one of the first books about

Its prize specimen The museum's most valued possession

ferocious mean, violent

teacher, but he loved the man; **there was in both a directness and plainness of conduct, an unquenchable desire for knowledge, and a congenial love of truth**." Dr. Baron reported that Jenner always referred to Mr. Hunter as "the dear man."

Still, Mr. Hunter was the strictest, most demanding person Jenner had ever known, or would know. Each day, he took his students to St. George's Hospital to show them patients with sicknesses the students had never seen before. Like all hospitals then, the wards were filthy, with used bandages piled up in the halls. Patients suffering from different diseases lay side by side, three, four, even five to a bed. In summer, flies buzzed around. In all seasons, the place smelled awful. Filthy conditions existed because of ignorance. Few eighteenth-century medical men knew that bacteria even existed, let alone caused sickness. Although Anton van Leeuwenhoek, a Dutch cloth merchant, had invented a simple microscope in the 1670s, its use spread slowly. English medical schools did not train students in the use of microscopes. Medical men spoke of "viruses," but the word had a different meaning than it does today. *Virus* simply meant "venom or poison"—nothing more.

To round out their education, Mr. Hunter sent his students to a small school run by his brother, William. There they learned how to deliver babies, studied the properties of various chemicals, and **dissected** dead bodies. The way the various organs of the human body actually worked and interacted with one another was still largely unknown. Since it was the general belief that humans were created in the image of God, the law banned the dissection of bodies in order to study anatomy, the body's structure. Only the bodies of executed criminals might go to the dissecting table. As a result, there were

....

there was in both a directness and plainness of conduct, an unquenchable desire for knowledge, and a congenial love of truth they were friendly with each other, curious to learn, and honest

dissected cut open

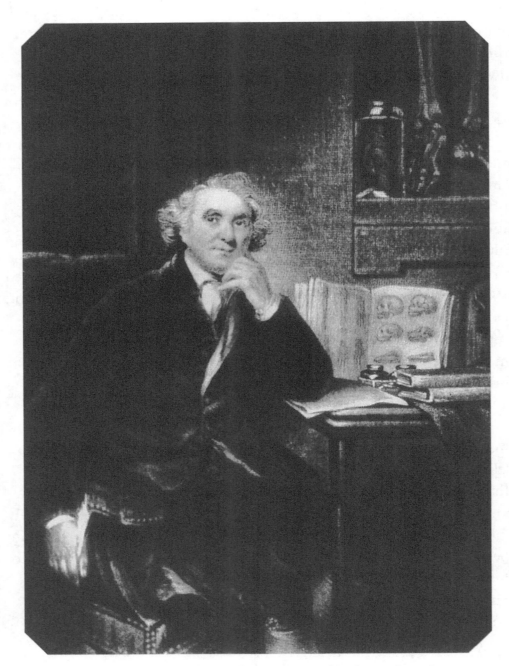

John Hunter, the greatest surgeon of the age, was Edward Jenner's teacher and friend. Hunter drummed a basic idea into his students' heads: "Try the experiment!" PHOTO COURTESY OF THE NATIONAL LIBRARY OF MEDICINE

never enough bodies available for study. To meet their needs, the Hunter brothers, like other medical men, sometimes hired thieves to rob graves in cemeteries.

Hunter's Teaching Methods

In return for their hard work, Mr. Hunter gave his students something more precious than gold. It was the gift of all great teachers. He taught them how to learn for themselves.

Once Jenner was **mulling over** a medical problem. Neither he nor Dr. Baron described that problem in their letters or other writings. All we know is that Jenner had thought about it **from every angle**, and still it puzzled him. Then Mr. Hunter **set him straight**. "Why think?" he wrote from London. "Why not try the experiment?"

Mr. Hunter did not recommend a particular experiment, or a method of experimenting, but the idea of experimentation itself. By that he meant devising ways to prove or disprove an idea, or to get nature to reveal something as yet unknown—a new truth—about itself. "Try the experiment" did not mean Jenner should stop thinking. Of course he should think, but only after he gathered enough facts, enough information, to allow him to think in new ways. In the spirit of the Age of Reason, Mr. Hunter taught his students that they could only get truth from facts. He urged them to **take nothing on faith**, to question authority, and to recheck their facts—often and in different ways. Once they were sure of these, they could think about what these meant and how to use them to help the sick.

Jenner learned well. After finishing his training in 1773, Mr.

---

mulling over thinking about

from every angle in every way he could

set him straight told him what to do

take nothing on faith demand proof

Hunter asked him to stay in London as his partner. Yet Jenner refused the honor. He wanted to go home to Berkeley.

Jenner as a Country Doctor

Edward Gardner, another friend of Jenner's, tells us in a letter that the young surgeon made a good impression on the local people back home. **Always on call**, Jenner charged according to the distance patients lived from the village, not the nature of their illness or the amount of time he spent with them. Jenner spoke softly to patients to avoid alarming them and their families. Like Mr. Ludlow, he traveled on horseback in all kinds of weather. Once he rode ten miles in a blizzard. Wind-driven snowflakes stung his face, making him wince in pain. It was so cold, he recalled, that he nearly froze to death. Before he could attend to his patient, a farmer, the man's family had to look after Jenner first. Only after Jenner thawed out could he do his job.

People liked Jenner, and he made friends easily. Edward Gardner left the only word-picture we have of him as an adult:

*His height was **rather under the middle size, his person was robust**, but active and well-formed. In his dress he was particularly neat, and everything about him showed a man intent and serious, and well prepared to meet the duties of his calling. . . . He was dressed in a blue coat and yellow buttons, buckskins, well-polished jockey boots, with handsome silver spurs, and he carried a smart whip with a silver handle. His hair, after the fashion of the times, was done up in a club, and he wore a*

....

Always on call Working whenever someone needed him

rather under the middle size, his person was robust *not very tall and a little heavy*

*broad-brimmed hat. . . . He was perfectly **unreserved, and free from all guile**. He carried his heart and his mind so openly, that all might read them.*

The two friends often rode to a favorite hilltop to admire the sunset. After dark, they visited a music club, where Jenner played the violin and flute. He also joined other country surgeons in **forming** a medical society. Every month or so, they met at the Ship Inn to discuss their **cases** over dinner and bottles of wine. In 1778 they had plenty to talk about.

....

unreserved, and free from all guile *friendly, open, and honest*

forming *creating*

cases *patients*

BEFORE YOU MOVE ON...

1. **Conclusions** Reread pages 48–50. People did not respect surgeons as much as doctors in the 1700s. Why not?

2. **Paraphrase** Reread page 55. What did John Hunter mean when he told Jenner to "try the experiment"?

LOOK AHEAD Read pages 58–67 to find out why women who milked cows did not get smallpox.

Return of an
Unwelcome Visitor

*Jenner looked for a new
way to fight smallpox.*

The Speckled Monster returned to the Berkeley area in 1778, after an absence of ten years. Like his fellow surgeons, Jenner did not know its true cause—and never would. Eighteenth-century medical men debated whether smallpox came from "putrid miasmas" (foul air) or from "**a vicious quality**" that a child got from its mother's blood while still in the womb. After the child was born, the disease supposedly struck when the body tried to **cleanse itself of the impurity**. Also, like his fellow surgeons, Jenner fought the disease in the usual way, with inoculation. Yet that made him uneasy.

Not only did Jenner know the risks of inoculation—that a person might die or spread the disease—he had personal reasons for disliking it. When he was eight, his brother had sent him to an inoculation stable. He never got over the frightful experience. For months afterward, it returned to him in nightmares. In 1821, two years before his death, Jenner **recalled how he had become sensitive to** certain sounds in that awful place. Although he had been there long, long ago, he told a family friend, the Reverend

....

a vicious quality a condition
cleanse itself of the impurity get rid of it
recalled how he had become sensitive to remembered how
he had learned to dislike

Worthington, he associated the experience with certain noises. Still "the horrible *click* of a spoon, knife, or fork falling upon a plate gives my brain a kind of death blow." In other words, the sound gave him a pounding headache. Jenner wondered: Might there be a better way of fighting the Speckled Monster?

Milkmaids Do Not Get Smallpox

The idea had first **crossed his mind** before 1770, during his stay with Mr. Ludlow. Like all country surgeons, Mr. Ludlow had milkmaids for patients, young women who made their living by milking dairy cows. While **calling at** a farm one day, Jenner had struck up a conversation with a pretty milkmaid. After a while the subject of smallpox came up. Had she ever been inoculated, he asked. No, she replied. Still, she did not fear the disease, since "I cannot take [get] smallpox, for I have had cowpox."

During visits to other farms, Jenner heard milkmaids sing as they went about their work:

> *"Where are you going, my pretty maid?*
> *I'm going a-milking, sir, she said.*
> *May I go with you, my pretty maid?*
> *You're kindly welcome, sir, she said.*
> *What is your father, my pretty maid?*
> *My father's a farmer, she said.*
> ***What is your fortune**, my pretty maid?*
> *My face is my fortune, she said."*

Milkmaids' faces were their fortunes, as the song said, because they

....

crossed his mind occurred to him

calling at visiting

What is your fortune *Do you have money*

had clear, smooth skin unmarked by smallpox scars, and could find husbands anytime they wished to marry. Although smallpox might tear through the rest of the community, it seemed to **pass them by**. And that, they said, was because they had already had "the cowpox."

Cowpox was a mild disease of cattle, found only in the British Isles and western Europe. Most likely, Jenner saw it on the milking cow his brother owned. (Many people, not just farmers, kept cows.) The infection appeared on an infected cow's **udder and teats** as red, swollen patches with bluish pustules at the center. The animal became restless and feverish, giving less milk. After a week or so, the symptoms passed and the cow recovered. Yet Jenner had never heard of a connection between cowpox and smallpox until the milkmaids mentioned it to him. When he told Mr. Ludlow of their claim, the surgeon called it **an ignorant superstition**. Later, John Hunter said the same thing. By then, in any case, other ideas filled Jenner's mind. He let the matter drop, **burying himself in** his studies.

Eight years later, however, as the smallpox epidemic of 1778 struck Berkeley and the surrounding countryside, Jenner recalled the milkmaid's words. The surgeon began to ask about cowpox during his rounds. Sure enough, the milkmaids he spoke to who had gotten cowpox remained free of smallpox, although they lived near people who were coming down with the dread disease. Farmers also repeated the folk saying: "If you want to marry a woman who will never be scarred by the pox, marry a milkmaid."

Did cowpox really prevent smallpox? Jenner wondered. If so, how? Was getting cowpox safer than having an inoculation? That could be an exciting discovery. But was it true? Mr. Hunter had taught him how to find out. Jenner must look carefully and gather his facts. Then, he must *try the experiment.*

....

pass them by leave them alone

udder and teats parts that hold the milk

an ignorant superstition a stupid and false belief

burying himself in concentrating on

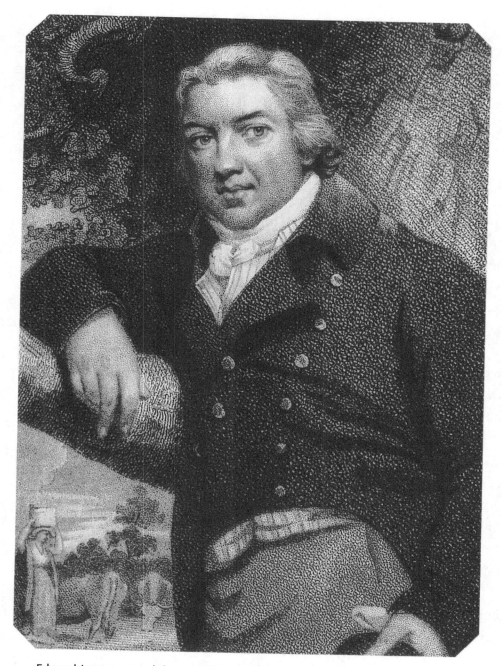

Edward Jenner around the year 1800. Notice the milkmaid in the background. Without these young women, he might never have gotten the idea that cowpox could protect against smallpox. PHOTO COURTESY OF THE NATIONAL LIBRARY OF MEDICINE

Cowpox and Its Mysterious Ways

*Jenner studied cowpox
and its symptoms.*

Jenner set out to study the symptoms of cowpox in humans. He began by visiting dairy farms to study the infection where it "lived." Milkmaids said that it was **horrid** to milk when the beast had their bag [udder] all broken out." Yet they did it anyhow, and without fear.

If a milkmaid happened to touch an infected udder or teat, droplets of pus might seep into any scratches or cuts on her hands. If so she would soon develop what seemed like the symptoms of smallpox inoculation, only far less severe. Pustules erupted on her fingers, hands, and wrists. **"The pulse is quickened,"** Jenner wrote in a notebook he kept, "and shiverings with general lassitude [fatigue] and **pains about the loins and limbs come on**. The head is painful . . . These symptoms, varying in their degree of violence, generally continue from day one to three or four. . . ." The discomfort passed by the sixth day, leaving the milkmaid good as new—with no pockmarks anywhere on her body. Cowpox is never deadly, either to animals or people.

Jenner knew nothing of immunity, let alone viruses. Three centuries ago, nobody had ever dreamed of them, much less seen any. Just how little he knew became evident to him toward the end of

---

horrid awful

The pulse is quickened The person's heart beats faster

pains about the loins and limbs come on the person's arms, chest, hips, and legs hurt

1778. Cowpox, he found, was a mysterious disease. It **seemed to have a mind of its own**, coming and going as it pleased. One year it would race through the dairies, infecting every cow. Then it would seem to vanish as suddenly as it had come. Years might pass without a single case. Then, just as suddenly, it would return for a short time. (Scientists still do not know why it vanishes, where it goes, or how it returns. Perhaps the virus does not "go" at all, but lies dormant— inactive—waiting for the right conditions, whatever they may be, to emerge. Perhaps it "hides" in another animal without causing an infection. Maybe it drifts in the air from place to place.)

Jenner questioned fellow surgeons at the medical clubs. Yes, they knew the farmers' sayings about milkmaids. Yet they did not believe a word of them. An animal disease protecting against a human disease! Why, if you believed that, they huffed, you might believe anything— like raw potatoes curing backaches and tobacco smoke helping shortness of breath, other pieces of folk "wisdom." The idea was so **much poppycock and fiddlesticks**!

Jenner needed to find out for himself. He persuaded a group of milkmaids who had had cowpox years before to let him inoculate them with pus from smallpox sufferers. None developed symptoms. To make sure he had done it right, he inoculated the same group again. Again, nothing! Yet when he inoculated another group of milkmaids, who had also had cowpox, some came down with the usual inoculation symptoms. He even heard of milkmaids elsewhere getting smallpox after having cowpox. "This," he wrote, "**gave a painful check to my fond and aspiring hopes**. But I resumed my labor with redoubled ardor."

Jenner could not leave the subject alone. Cowpox as a possible way to prevent smallpox was all he wanted to talk about during those

....

seemed to have a mind of its own was unpredictable

much poppycock and fiddlesticks ridiculous, silly

gave a painful check to my fond and aspiring hopes disappointed me

evenings around the dinner table with fellow surgeons. Dr. Baron recalled that he became a pest, although Dr. Baron did not use that word. Jenner talked so much that surgeons gritted their teeth whenever he entered a room. Finally, Dr. Baron said, "It became so distasteful to his companions . . . that they threatened to expel him if he continued to harass them with so unprofitable a subject." Jenner took the hint and changed the subject—at least around them.

Cowpox still came and went as unpredictably as ever. Meanwhile, Jenner kept making his rounds, making his observations, and asking his questions. Yet he could not figure out why some cowpox sufferers got inoculation symptoms or even the disease itself, and others got nothing.

The years passed. In 1788 he married Catherine Kingscote, a landowner's daughter. In 1792, the University of St. Andrews in Scotland gave him a doctor's degree in medicine—without Jenner ever taking a test. All he had to do was send a cash gift and letters of recommendation from two doctors. The doctors said they knew him well, and that he had "attended a complete course of **lectures in the several branches of Medicine**" during his time with Mr. Hunter. From then on he signed his name Edward Jenner, M.D.—Doctor of Medicine. In doing so, he joined the **handful of** English surgeons who became doctors.

In his spare time, Jenner studied the habits of birds, a favorite hobby, and sent specimens to Mr. Hunter for his museum. The older man loved hearing from his friend. "Dear Jenner," he wrote, "I do not know anyone I would sooner write to than you: I do not know anybody I am so much obliged to."

Jenner also studied angina pectoris, a disease that causes severe chest pains. He had the chance to **do autopsies on** two people who

----

lectures in the several branches of Medicine many different medical classes

handful of few

do autopsies on cut open and examine

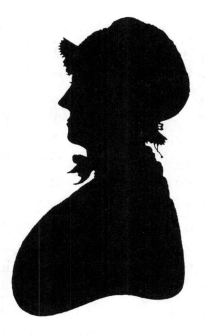

A silhouette of Catherine Jenner, the doctor's wife, done during their early married life. PHOTO IN AUTHOR'S COLLECTION

had died of this disease; he never said who they were or how he got the chance. Anyhow, he discovered that angina sufferers always had the blood vessels of their heart clogged with fat—probably from the fatty foods they ate, Jenner believed. He reasoned—correctly—that fat blocked the flow of blood, bringing on fatal heart attacks. In the eighteenth century, any type of heart disease was incurable. Since Mr. Hunter had angina, Jenner hid his findings, for fear of putting him under further stress. The "dear man" died of heart failure in 1793.

How Jenner Solves the Cowpox Riddle

That same year, Jenner solved the riddle of cowpox. **The solution came to him** in the barn behind his house. Like most villagers, he

....

The solution came to him He solved the problem

kept a cow to provide his family with fresh milk; although he sometimes milked it himself, a servant usually did the job. Cowpox had returned to Berkeley, and the doctor's animal was just getting over it.

Late one night, Jenner went to the barn to tidy it up. Everything was quiet, apart from his cow's lazy munching on her straw. It had been a long day. After finishing his work in the barn, Jenner sat on a wooden box for a moment before going to bed. He sat motionless, just **bathing in the delicious silence**. With his mind and body relaxed, the answer seemed to arrive on its own. It came not from any new facts he found, but from those he had been thinking about for years. Only now they **fell into place** in his mind in exactly the right way.

Years later, Jenner recalled that he suddenly realized "that the virus [poison] of cowpox **was liable to undergo progressive changes** in the cow." In other words, he theorized that the matter in the pustules must vary in strength over the course of the infection. At the outset, he thought, the "virus" had not grown strong enough to prevent a reaction to a smallpox inoculation. But with time, it "gained in power," as he put it, thus increasing its ability to protect against smallpox. Finally, in its last stages, it might produce mild symptoms of cowpox but offered no protection against the Speckled Monster. Cowpox, then, was effective to prevent against smallpox only if a person got the "virus" at the height of the disease in an infected animal.

Although Jenner was on the right track, he could not really explain why. Modern immunologists explain the protective effect of pus from cowpox infections as a result of the close similarity between the cowpox virus and the virus that causes smallpox. Cowpox virus is not

....

bathing in the delicious silence enjoying the quiet

fell into place became clear

was liable to undergo progressive changes was likely to change

as dangerous to humans as the smallpox virus, and being exposed to it causes relatively mild symptoms. But it is similar enough that the antibodies and T cells made by the immune system of a person exposed to cowpox will also react with and destroy smallpox. As a cowpox infection develops in an infected cow, the amount of virus present in the animal at first increases. But after about two weeks the cow's immune system succeeds in destroying the virus. Thus the amount of virus to be found in the cow's pus will at first increase and then decline, and that is why it is important to choose the best time to collect material from the animal in order to get the maximum amount of virus—and the strongest protective effect. **If the disease takes hold anyhow**, it is because the person's immune system has been compromised—weakened—by poor health or in other ways.

Jenner had to prove that his **theory** was correct—that cowpox pus taken at full strength protected against smallpox. To do that, he had to *try the experiment!* Yet cowpox refused to cooperate—as usual. In the fall of 1793, it suddenly vanished from the Berkeley dairies. But Jenner knew it would return, and he set to work so that when it did, he would be ready.

....

If the disease takes hold anyhow If the person cannot fight the disease

theory idea

BEFORE YOU MOVE ON...

1. Assumption Milkmaids rarely got smallpox. What did people assume about them? How do you know?

2. Summarize Reread pages 66–67. How did cowpox protect against smallpox?

LOOK AHEAD Read pages 68–76 to find out if Jenner's experiment was successful.

The *G*reat Experiment

*Jenner used smallpox to
create the smallpox vaccine.*

*J*enner set up his experiment carefully. Getting pus at the height of
an infection would not be a problem. Once cowpox returned, he
would have plenty of animals to choose from. Still, he knew, cowpox
was bound to vanish again. Jenner had to think of the future. If his
experiment worked, he would need a way to give people resistance to
smallpox even after cowpox disappeared from dairies. To do that, he
decided to **adopt** the "arm-to-arm" method. He would take pus from
a cow and scratch it into the arm of a person. When pustules formed,
he would scratch pus from them into the arm of someone else, and so
on. Thus, Jenner would eventually transfer cowpox not from animals
to people but from one person to another.

Three years later, in the spring of 1796, cowpox returned to
Berkeley. Jenner's chance had come. One day, Sarah Nelmes, nineteen,
stuck her finger on a thorn before milking Blossom, a cow with large
pustules on her udder. (Blossom became famous, and her **hide** is
preserved in the library of St. George's Hospital.) Pustules soon
appeared on Sarah's fingers and wrists. When Jenner saw them, he
realized that she had cowpox. Now he must try the experiment!

"I selected a healthy boy, about eight years old, for the purpose of

---

was bound to vanish would probably disappear

adopt use

hide skin

inoculation with cowpox," Jenner wrote in his notebook. "The matter was taken from a sore on the hand of a dairymaid, who was infected by her master's cows, and it was inserted, on the 14th of May, 1796, into the arm of the boy by two **[incisions]**, each about half an inch long." The only record we have of the boy's name, James Phipps, comes from a letter Jenner wrote his friend Edward Garner.

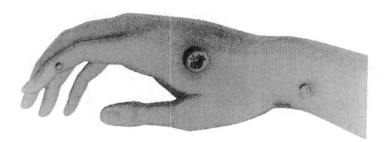

The cowpox pustules of milkmaid Sarah Nelmes. Jenner used pus from her hand for his first vaccination. PHOTO COURTESY OF THE NATIONAL LIBRARY OF MEDICINE

James's parents were day laborers who had done odd jobs for the Jenner family for years. Jenner did not say how he convinced them to let him experiment on their son. Did he reason with them, assuring them that cowpox was safe? Did he tell them that the experiment could help their son escape smallpox and possibly help all humanity? Perhaps he simply ordered these poor people to bring their son to him—or else he would see that they never worked in Berkeley again? This is hard to imagine; there is no record of Jenner's ever threatening, let alone harming, another person. We may never know how he persuaded them.

Later, some medical men accused Jenner of using James as **a guinea pig**. In other words, they claimed he **deliberately risked the youngster's life** without thought or care for his welfare.

Jenner's aim was to help James, not to hurt him. Jenner knew

....

[incisions] [cuts]

a guinea pig an experiment

deliberately risked the youngster's life purposely put the boy in danger

milkmaids had gotten cowpox and always recovered. Yet he did not know how a child would react to cowpox, or the "right" dosage of pus to give to him. That is where the risk lay. Even so, Jenner thought there was little to lose and everything to gain. He was trying to protect James from an awful disease. As we have seen, children were more likely to get smallpox than adults; English children usually got it by the age of seven. Thus, before long, the boy was almost certain to **have a run-in** with the Speckled Monster. Even if the experiment failed, James would not be any worse off than before, since so far as Jenner knew, nobody had ever died of cowpox. If it succeeded, Jenner believed James would gain the same protection against smallpox that milkmaids seemed to have, without the danger and pain of inoculation in the ordinary way.

Jenner's notebook records:

> *On the seventh day he [James] complained of **uneasiness** at the axilla [armpits], and on the ninth he became a little **chilly**, lost his appetite, and had a slight headache. During the whole of this day he was [uncomfortable], and spent the night with some degree of restlessness, but on the following day was perfectly well.*

Soon afterward, James developed pustules, which later became scabs and fell off. In other words, he came down with the symptoms of cowpox and then recovered. **So far so good.** The real test came next. Smallpox had broken out in the Berkeley area again. On July 1, Jenner inoculated James with pus taken from the arm of a man with a raging case of the disease. "Several slight punctures and incisions were made on both his arms," Jenner wrote, "and the matter was carefully inserted, but no disease followed." James showed no ill effects

....

have a run-in be infected

uneasiness discomfort

chilly cold, feverish

So far so good. This was a good sign.

whatsoever. In years to come, Jenner would introduce smallpox material into James twenty times, just to make sure. Each gave the same reaction—that is, no reaction at all. James did not come down with smallpox. Thrilled with the results, Jenner built a cottage for James near his own house. Today the house is the Jenner Museum.

Jenner conducted more experiments during a twin outbreak of cowpox and smallpox in 1798. He began by giving cowpox to Hanna Excell, described as "a healthy girl of seven years old." When cowpox symptoms appeared on her, he injected four other children with matter from Hanna's pustules. This group included "one-and-a-half-year-old Robert F. Jenner," proof of his father's faith in his method. Each time he inoculated someone with cowpox, Jenner followed up with a smallpox inoculation. The children simply would not "take the pox." As with James Phipps, they resisted smallpox without ever having had the disease.

The Effects of Jenner's Discovery

Jenner took pride in his experiments, particularly the first one, with Phipps. "The joy I felt," he wrote Edward Gardner, "was so excessive that I sometimes found myself in a kind of reverie"—a wonderful daydream.

A religious man, he felt that God had chosen him for a sacred mission. Cowpox inoculation was the blessing that humanity had been waiting for. And he, Edward Jenner, M.D., would teach the world how to use it. He explained: "The **annihilation** of smallpox, the **most dreadful scourge** of the human species, must be the final result of this practice."

....

annihilation end

most dreadful scourge worst disease

71

The annihilation of smallpox. Let these words sink into your mind. They are more important than they may at first seem. **In them we hear the stirrings of a new era in human history**, an era of hope based on scientific knowledge. Until then, people had thought of disease as inevitable, as much a part of being human as eating and sleeping. Disease was just something that "came"—something you had to endure, perhaps even die from.

Not anymore. Starting with Jenner's experiments, the idea that humans are not helpless against disease became a proven truth. Now for the first time ever, it truly seemed possible to eliminate a disease. Conquering the Speckled Monster was the first step. If humanity could do that, then it might do anything. It might, perhaps, annihilate all diseases.

Toward the end of 1798, Jenner described his experiments and their results in a pamphlet titled *An Inquiry into the Causes and Effects of the Variolae Vaccinae . . . Known by the Name of the Cow Pox.* Two other pamphlets followed: *Further Observations on the Variolae Vaccinae, or Cow-Pox* (1799), and *Continuation of Facts and Observations Relative to Variolae Vaccinae* (1800). The Latin word for cow is *vacca; Variolae vaccinae* is simply "the pox taken from the cow."

The 1798 pamphlet **circulated widely** among medical men in England. Injecting cowpox seemed safer, and more effective, than old-style inoculation. To highlight the fact that Jenner's method differed from inoculation, in 1803 Mr. Richard Dunning, surgeon, called injecting people with cowpox matter "vaccination." The name **stuck**. Seventy years later, the great French chemist, Louis Pasteur, would honor Jenner by calling any inoculation that produces immunity to any disease a "vaccination." Pasteur called the matter used in a vaccination a "vaccine."

....

In them we hear the stirrings of a new era in human history
These words mean that the world has changed forever

circulated widely was well known

stuck became popular

AN

INQUIRY

INTO

THE CAUSES AND EFFECTS

OF

THE VARIOLÆ VACCINÆ,

A DISEASE

DISCOVERED IN SOME OF THE WESTERN COUNTIES OF ENGLAND,

PARTICULARLY

GLOUCESTERSHIRE,

AND KNOWN BY THE NAME OF

THE COW POX.

———————

BY EDWARD JENNER, M.D. F.R.S. &c.

———————

———— QUID NOBIS CERTIUS IPSIS
SENSIBUS ESSE POTEST, QUO VERA AC FALSA NOTEMUS.

LUCRETIUS.

————————

London:

PRINTED, FOR THE AUTHOR,

BY SAMPSON LOW, N°. 7, BERWICK STREET, SOHO:

AND SOLD BY LAW, AVE-MARIA LANE; AND MURRAY AND HIGHLEY, FLEET STREET.

———

1798.

Title page of Jenner's first pamphlet describing his cowpox experiments. This pamphlet became a sensation, encouraging other medical men to duplicate his work. PHOTO COURTESY OF THE NATIONAL LIBRARY OF MEDICINE

Friends and Enemies

*Many people did
not trust Jenner's vaccine.*

English doctors flooded Jenner with requests for cowpox vaccine
to use in their own experiments. He usually sent it in **a goose quill**
or in a glass vial containing a string attached to the end of a needle
that had been passed through a pustule. The cowpox virus could
not survive outside a host for more than a few days. If the doctors
were lucky and the virus survived, the vaccination "took" when they
scratched the vaccine into a patient's arm. The patient developed
the symptoms of cowpox. Then they used the arm–to–arm method
to vaccinate others.

Yet vaccination also had its enemies. As with inoculation earlier,
there were those who saw it as **a rejection of** God's will. Dr. William
Rowley, of Oxford, called it "a daring violation of our holy religion."
The Reverend Dr. Squirrel asked Sunday school classes why Moses'
mother had hidden him in the **bulrushes** along the Nile River. The
children were supposed to answer: "Because they wanted to vaccinate
him." The Reverend Thomas R. Malthus went further. He praised
smallpox as a gift sent by a loving God to **hold down** the number of
poor people. Eliminating it would only allow poverty to spread,
making the poor more miserable than ever, he claimed.

....

a goose quill the hollow part of a feather
a rejection of going against
bulrushes grass-like leaves
hold down decrease

Opponents attacked Jenner personally, too, calling him a liar, a fool, and the devil's tool. Some medical men had **grown** rich from giving inoculations. They feared vaccination might hurt their business. Others were so set in their ideas that they could not imagine ever being wrong. Why, they said, vaccination was more dangerous than inoculation. Yes, inoculation might kill a patient, which was bad enough. Vaccination stole their humanity because the vaccine "bovinized" them—turned them into cattle. One doctor claimed to know of a girl changed into a "brutish creature" by vaccination. She "coughed like a cow, and had grown hairy over her body." Another described an "ox–faced boy" who **bellowed** at the sight of strangers.

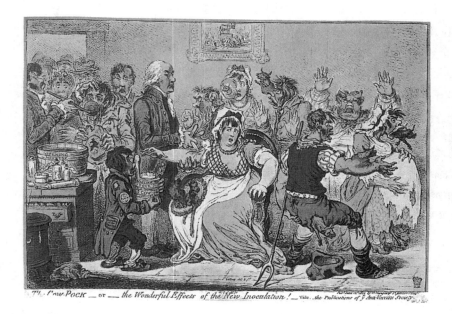

Th. Cow Pock — or — the Wonderful Effects of the New Inoculation! — vide. the Publications of y.e Anti Vaccine Society.

Not everyone thought vaccination a good idea. In this famous cartoon of 1802, James Gillray showed that vaccination was downright dangerous. Others, however, thought it foolish to believe that vaccination would cause little cows to pop out all over a patient's body. PHOTO IN AUTHOR'S COLLECTION

....

grown become

bellowed made loud noises

The Anti-Vaccine Society of London hired artists to spread its message. Its best-known work was a cartoon of 1802 by James Gillray. Titled "The Cow-Pock, or, the Wonderful Effects of the New Inoculation!" it shows Jenner vaccinating a woman with "**pock hot from ye cow**." Patients vaccinated moments earlier are standing nearby. They do not look happy. Miniature cows spring from their mouths, cheeks, noses, ears, and arms. One unhappy woman is giving birth to a calf!

Most people **dismissed this as nonsense**. Dr. John Ring, of London, saw no harm in vaccination. He noted that people eat steak, and children drink cows' milk, without being bovinized. Why, then, should a drop of vaccine change them? It should not; so he continued to vaccinate. The Reverend Rowland Hill, a respected churchman, also vaccinated. He would stand in his pulpit on Sundays, after the sermon, to say, "I am ready to vaccinate tomorrow morning as many children as you choose; and if you wish them to escape that horrible disease, the smallpox, you will bring them!" Slowly, **the tide was turning against superstition**.

....

pock hot from ye cow fresh pus from a cow

dismissed this as nonsense did not believe it

the tide was turning against superstition people were starting to believe that vaccination was not dangerous

BEFORE YOU MOVE ON...

1. **Sequence** Reread pages 69–71. Jenner's experiment with cowpox was successful. Describe his experiment.

2. **Argument** Reread pages 74–75. What reasons did people give for arguing against Jenner's vaccination?

LOOK AHEAD Read pages 77–88 to find out how Jenner's vaccine affected the rest of the world.

Dr. Jenner's Gift to the World

*The smallpox vaccine
reached countries around the world.*

Vaccination knew no boundaries or politics. News of its successes in England spread quickly. Although nearly all Europe was then at war with France, nothing blocked this important news. French, German, Spanish, Dutch, Italian, and Latin translations of Jenner's 1798 pamphlet appeared soon after its publication. **Cooperation not only seemed morally right, but** was also practical. **The Speckled Monster played no favorites.** Wars come and go. Time turns enemies into friends. But there was one war that never ended, and one enemy that never changed. The Speckled Monster threatened everyone and knew no boundaries. No nation could be safe while it **ravaged** another.

Vaccination reached Austria first. When Jean de Carro, a leading doctor, wrote Jenner for a vaccine sample, Jenner sent it gladly. De Carro knew high officials in the Austrian government. To make sure the vaccine reached him safely, they created an early version of the Pony Express. Once it arrived at a Dutch seaport, special riders carried it nonstop to Austria. The results were so

....

Cooperation not only seemed morally right, but
Vaccinating people was the right thing to do and

The Speckled Monster played no favorites. Smallpox
affected everyone.

ravaged destroyed

promising that de Carro recommended vaccination to doctors in Poland, Hungary, Russia, and Italy.

Alexander I, emperor of Russia, wanted his subjects vaccinated. On his orders, every town formed a vaccination committee to do the job. To make sure things ran smoothly, he formed an Imperial Medical Police to keep watch over the committees. The emperor even changed the name of the first child vaccinated to "Vaccinoff" and brought him to the capital in a golden coach. In all, Russian doctors vaccinated nearly 2 million children. His Majesty sent Jenner a valuable diamond ring as a reward.

Religious **processions** in Italy carried "the blessed vaccine" through city streets. Priests led their people right to the vaccinators' doors behind golden crosses and holy banners. To show vaccination's safety, doctors had orphan children who had been vaccinated share beds with smallpox victims. None got sick. In **rural areas**, where there were few doctors, Catholic priests gave vaccinations themselves, in churches, beneath the statues of saints.

Despite France's war with England, the French leader, Napoleon Bonaparte, sent Dr. Aubert, of Paris, to England to study vaccination from English doctors. The English welcomed him. Although Jenner did not meet him, he was glad the Frenchman had come to learn and do good. "The sciences are never at war," he said.

When Dr. Aubert returned to France, Napoleon ordered vaccinations for all his soldiers who had not had smallpox. The English military welcomed that action; they did not want French war prisoners carrying smallpox into their army. Napoleon admired few people, and these were soldiers like himself. He hated doctors. Whenever he met one, he would **open with** the question: "How many patients have you killed in your practice?" Yet Jenner was special.

....

promising good
processions parades
rural areas country places
open with begin by asking

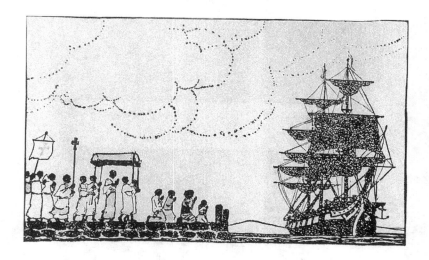

The king of Spain sent a fleet to spread vaccination around the globe. In this picture, Catholics welcome a Spanish ship with a religious procession.
PHOTO COURTESY OF THE WORLD HEALTH ORGANIZATION

When Jenner wrote asking Napoleon to free some English prisoners, he could not turn him down. "Jenner!" he snorted, "Ah, I can refuse nothing to that man."

Vaccination **crossed the border** from France to Spain. King Carlos IV sent a fleet to the New World, not to fight, but to bring vaccination to Spain's colonies. He called it the Royal Vaccination **Expedition**. Since it would take about ten weeks to cross the Atlantic Ocean, there was only one way to maintain a fresh vaccine supply. The expedition's **flagship** carried twenty-two boys, aged three to nine, taken from an orphanage. They had never had smallpox. Just before the fleet sailed, Francisco Xavier de Balmis, its chief surgeon, vaccinated two children. Every week thereafter, he vaccinated two others with pus taken from those vaccinated the week before, creating, in effect, a living chain of donors. The **fleet** visited Puerto Rico, Cuba, Mexico, and South America. Then, with a new group of children aboard, it crossed the Pacific Ocean to the Philippine Islands and China. The expedition lasted three years, from 1803 to 1806.

....

crossed the border spread
Expedition Journey, Voyage
flagship main ship
fleet ships

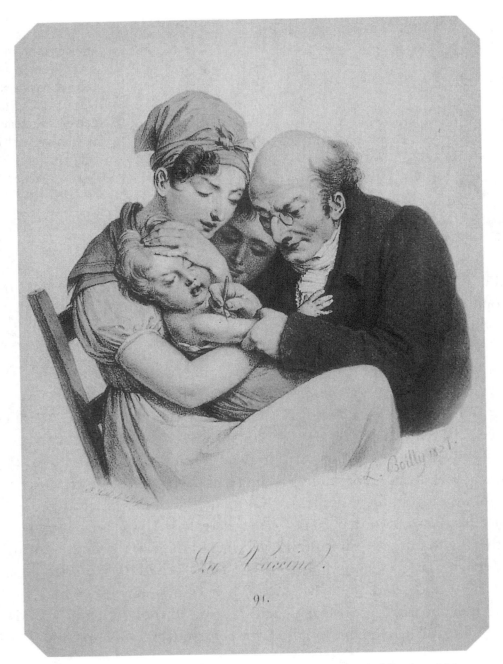

In 1827, French artist Louis-Léopold Boilly painted a mother holding her child as a doctor administers the vaccine. Especially vulnerable to smallpox, children were vaccinated as early as possible. Photo courtesy of the National Library of Medicine

Before it ended, its doctors vaccinated 230,000 children.

Dr. Benjamin Waterhouse, of Boston, became the American Edward Jenner. A daring experimenter, inspired by Jenner's writings, he began in 1800 by vaccinating four of his own sons, then tested them with smallpox pus. "The only reason why I tested my own children with Small Pox," he explained, "was not to satisfy myself, but **the public**. I did it, with regard to my own children, to show my entire confidence in the practice." When they showed no ill effects, he repeated the experiment on nineteen orphans sent to him by the Boston Board of Health. These children also did well. Finally, to prove that the smallpox pus still had its full strength, he took an awful risk: He inoculated two orphan boys who had never had cowpox or smallpox. Both got smallpox, but survived with scars on their faces. No proper scientist would do such a dangerous thing today. Nevertheless, Waterhouse proved to Americans, beyond any doubt, that vaccination protected against the Speckled Monster.

Waterhouse reported his findings to Thomas Jefferson. Excited by the news, the third president of the United States lost no time in having his family and slaves vaccinated at Monticello, his Virginia plantation. The president also sent army surgeons to vaccinate the Indians in the Louisiana Territory, purchased from France in 1803. Unfortunately, before the program **really got underway** money ran out, with tragic results.

Effect of Smallpox on Native Americans

As in colonial times, smallpox tore through Native American communities. From 1836 to 1840, it **ravaged** the western tribes. A

---

the public to satisfy everyone
really got underway began
ravaged killed many people in

steamboat accidentally carried it to the Mandan, who lived in large villages along the Missouri River in North Dakota. Lacking any immunity, the population of one village fell from two thousand to under forty in less than a month. Horrified at how the disease was **disfiguring them, and racked with pain, people committed suicide**. Artist George Catlin watched them. "They destroyed themselves with their knives, with their guns, and by dashing their

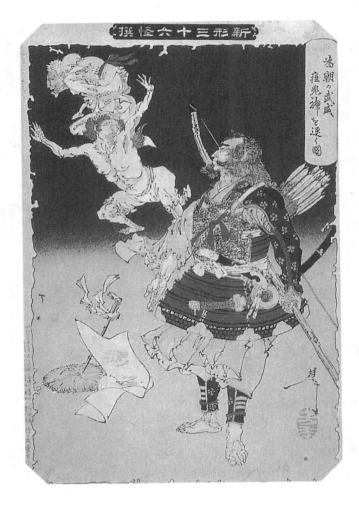

This nineteenth-century woodcut shows the Japanese archer Tametomo victorious over smallpox, which is presented as an evil person.
PHOTO COURTESY OF THE WORLD HEALTH ORGANIZATION

....
disfiguring them, and racked with pain, people committed suicide changing the way they looked and causing them pain, people killed themselves

brains out by leaping **head-foremost** from a thirty-foot ledge of rocks in front of their village." Scenes like this took place in every Mandan village, and the tribe never recovered. From the Mandan villages, smallpox spread to the buffalo-hunting tribes of the Great Plains. Among these were the Lakota, Cheyenne, Crow, Pawnee, Comanche, Blackfeet, Snake, and Arikara.

Since the Plains Indians got the disease and most whites did not, they reasoned that the strangers had introduced it to get rid of them and take their lands. Whites, they said, had an invisible **ally**, a demon Indians called the Smallpox Rider. The demon was always by the strangers' side, always ready to fight their battles. "I am one with the White People," they believed the Smallpox Rider said. "Sometimes I travel ahead of them, and sometimes behind. But I am always their companion and you will find me in their camps and their houses. I bring Death."

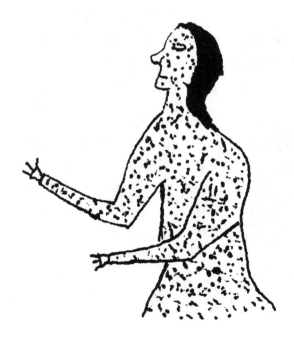

In the 1800s, Plains Indian tribes like the Oglala Sioux painted "winter counts," records of the year's main events, on pieces of tanned buffalo hide. This one shows a man covered with smallpox pustules. The disease decimated the Great Plains tribes, making it easier for white settlers to take their lands. PHOTO IN AUTHOR'S COLLECTION

head-foremost headfirst

ally friend, partner

An elder of the Peigan nation named Saukamappee lived through the Speckled Monster's attack. His band had raided enemies, the Shoshone Indians, only to find their camp filled with the dead and dying. Shocked, the raiders fled, taking a few Shoshone blankets and tents. They had no idea that these held bits of scab shed by disease victims. So, without meaning to, the raiders brought the Speckled Monster to their own families. Saukamappee told a white fur trader what happened next:

> *"This dreadful disease broke out in our camp, and spread from one tent to another as if the Bad Spirit carried it. We had no belief that one man could give it to another, any more than a wounded man could give his wound to another. . . . About one third of us died, but in some of the camps there were tents in which everyone died. When at length it left us, and we moved about to find our people,* **it was no longer with the song and the dance; but with tears, shrieks, and howlings of despair for those who would never return to us.** *. . . We believed the Good Spirit had* **forsaken** *us, and allowed the Bad Spirit to become our master."*

Smallpox reduced the population of the Great Plains tribes about a fourth—more than thirty thousand people—within five years. Later outbreaks took fewer lives, because there were fewer lives to take. Yet the damage was already done. In the end, the disease helped break Native American resistance to the whites' takeover of the Far West.

....

it was no longer with the song and the dance; but with tears, shrieks, and howlings of despair for those who would never return to us *we did not search with joy; but with tears, screams, and cries for those who had died*

forsaken *left, abandoned*

Jenner's Last Days

Jenner became world famous.

By 1805, Edward Jenner, at fifty-six, was world famous. Offers came to Jenner from London. If he would move there, a group of doctors promised to help him get rich by vaccinating the wealthy. Jenner **turned them down**. By moving to that noisy, bustling city, **"What stock should I add to my little fund of happiness?"** he asked. All he needed for a happy life he already had at Berkeley: family, friends, everyone's love and respect. In short, he would rather live modestly and do good than **roll in money among strangers**.

Jenner still worked hard—very hard. He spent each morning writing "till I am grown as crooked as a cow's horn." Letters piled up on his writing table, some of them from critics. Vaccination, they wrote, did not work; in fact, it was deadly. They knew, for they had vaccinated patients arm to arm, only to have them die of diseases like syphilis. Politely, Jenner explained that although transferring vaccine from one person to another protected against smallpox, a vaccine donor could pass on another contagious disease. Had Jenner known that bacteria cause disease, he might have added another caution. Vaccinating without first disinfecting the instruments and the

....

turned them down did not accept their offers

"What stock should I add to my little fund of happiness?"
"How would moving to London make me happier?"

roll in money among strangers become rich and live with people he did not know

vaccination site would allow infections to enter the bloodstream.

Most letters, however, came from fellow doctors who wanted his advice on vaccination. Travelers asked him to write Napoleon for permission to pass through France without fear of arrest. Others praised Jenner and his work for humanity. President Jefferson, an admirer, wrote to say that "**Yours is the comfortable reflection that mankind can never forget that you have lived.** Future nations will know by history only that the loathsome smallpox had existed and by you had been **extirpated**."

Nearly every scientific society in Europe and America made Jenner a member. Universities gave him honorary degrees. Germans celebrated the day he vaccinated James Phipps, May 14, as a holiday. In 1813 even Oxford University recognized his achievement. Although some professors still looked down on him as "a mere surgeon" who had bought a medical degree, the university awarded him the degree of Doctor of Medicine. Every honor and request called for a written reply. Jenner had become, as he put it, the "vaccine clerk to the world."

Jenner's Good Deeds

Yet he never forgot his duty to **those less fortunate**. Busy as Jenner was, in the early 1800s, he set aside one day a week to vaccinate free of charge those who could not afford to pay.

Before dawn, rain or shine, country people began to appear at his front gate. Most were women holding babies in their arms or leading toddlers by the hand. Sometimes as many as three hundred came. As they arrived, a servant had them line up by the door of a stone cottage

---

Yours is the comfortable reflection that mankind can never forget that you had lived. People will never forget you.

extirpated destroyed

those less fortunate the poor

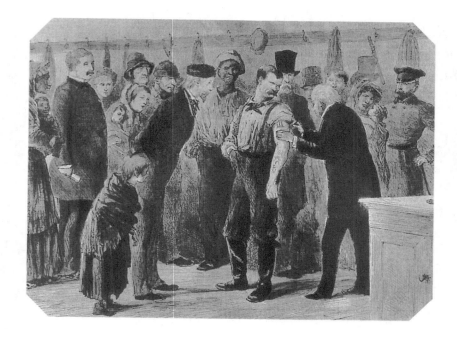

Vaccinating the Poor, a painting done by the artist Sol Eytinge, Jr., about the year 1873. By then, most European countries offered free vaccination as a public health measure. Photo courtesy of the National Library of Medicine

in the garden. Jenner called this cottage the Temple of Vaccinia. It still stands. On vaccination days, he thanked God for the "blessing" of allowing him to save so many from the Speckled Monster.

The years **sped by**—happy, busy, productive years, broken only by the death of his wife, Catherine, in 1815. Already, Jenner was beginning to feel **his age**. His eyesight grew dimmer, his hands trembled, and his bones ached on rainy days. Jenner knew he **had more time behind him than ahead of him**.

And so he did. On January 25, 1823, a blood vessel burst in his brain. The next day, Edward Jenner died, four months short of his seventy-fourth birthday. James Phipps stood in the crowd of mourners during the funeral service in Berkeley church. Jenner's tombstone bears these words:

....

sped by passed quickly

his age old

had more time behind him than ahead of him was approaching death

*Within this tomb **hath** found a resting place*
The great physician of the human race—
Immortal Jenner! *Whose gigantic mind*
Brought life and health to more than half mankind.

No stone ever had truer words carved into it.

....

hath *Jenner has*
Immortal Jenner! *Jenner will always be remembered!*

BEFORE YOU MOVE ON...

1. **Conclusions** How did the smallpox vaccine unite countries around the world?

2. **Comparisons** Reread pages 85–86. People had mixed reactions to vaccination. What were they?

LOOK AHEAD Read pages 89–96 to find out why doctors changed Jenner's vaccination method.

The Final Victory

*Doctors and scientists
continued to improve the vaccine.*

Jenner was gone, but his work continued. In the years after his death, one country after another banned inoculation as too dangerous. In its place, European governments ordered children vaccinated before they attended school for the first time; the state paid the cost. This was an important development. For the first time in history, governments ordered entire nations to take **a health precaution**.

Although vaccination protected against smallpox, the arm–to–arm method could spread other diseases, as Jenner had noted. Italian doctors abandoned the arm–to–arm method in 1843. In its place, they devised a new method. After shaving the belly of a calf, they scratched vaccine into the skin in several places. When pustules formed, they led the calf from house to house, vaccinating children on their own doorstep. However, using the same instrument on one person after another also spread diseases other than smallpox. That problem was solved by the 1890s, when **the mass production of sterile, throwaway needles began**.

In the twentieth century, laboratories began freeze-drying cowpox vaccine to preserve it for later use. By then, however, it was no longer

....

a health precaution action to prevent sickness

the mass production of sterile, throwaway needles began
needles were made that were thrown away after one use

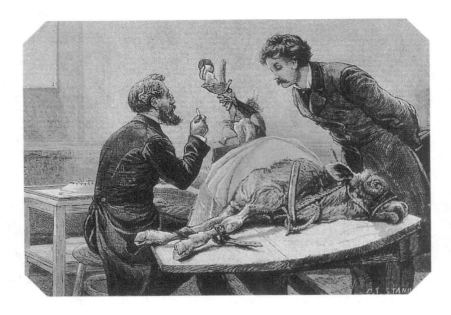

Before scientists learned how to preserve vaccine, they brought a cow infected with cowpox to each patient's house and drew pus from a pustule that seemed to be at the right stage of development. Photo courtesy of the World Health Organization

the same virus Jenner had used. Scientists believe the **original virus mutated** into something new, called vaccinia. Nobody knows how, why, or when this happened. However it happened, vaccinia also prevents assaults from the Speckled Monster.

Scientists gradually began to vaccinate against diseases other than smallpox. **A key breakthrough** came in 1885, when Louis Pasteur made a vaccine to prevent rabies. This painful disease, dreaded since ancient times, is caused by a virus that gets into the saliva of warm-blooded animals like dogs, cats, squirrels, and bats. The virus drives the host animal into a frenzy of biting, and thus new victims are infected. Today, thanks to vaccination, science has **eradicated** rabies in much of the world.

With Pasteur, however, vaccination took a giant step forward. Jenner had used material from an animal disease to protect against a human disease. Pasteur and his followers made vaccines of an entirely

....

original virus mutated first virus changed

A key breakthrough An important discovery

eradicated completely removed

different kind. Instead of material from an animal with a related disease, today's vaccines are made of chemically weakened or killed forms of actual bacteria and viruses that cause disease in humans. When vaccinated with one of these, the patient's immune system reacts naturally, as if the disease had invaded the body. The immune system goes to work and produces the antibodies reacting specifically with those bacteria or viruses. Should **the disease strike** later, the immune system is now **primed** to resist it.

Medical researchers continued to make progress. As of the year 2000, the development of vaccines against more than twenty infectious diseases has allowed people to live healthier, more productive lives. We now have vaccines against such **old-time killers** as influenza, whooping cough, meningitis, diphtheria, typhoid, yellow fever, bubonic plague, measles, hepatitis B, and mumps. In 1996 the World Health Organization of the United Nations estimated that, without vaccination, these diseases would have claimed at least 15 million lives each year. Moreover, we are about to see humanity's victory over polio. Soon, vaccination may finally eradicate this viral disease, which has killed, paralyzed, or crippled countless people over the centuries.

Status of Smallpox in the 20ᵗʰ Century

Yet the struggle against contagious diseases is far from over. Just as our immune systems have ways of defeating invading bacteria and viruses, these microbes can find ways to defeat the immune system. Viruses and bacteria are constantly mutating. Although most mutations do not help them survive, some do. Some prevent the immune system

---

the disease strike the person get the disease
primed ready, prepared
old-time killers diseases that once killed people

from recognizing them as dangerous. HIV, the virus that causes AIDS, attacks the immune system itself. Scientists think HIV began as a mild disease of African chimpanzees, then **found its way into** hunters who had been exposed to infected blood. The hunters then spread the disease to their families and other villagers through sexual contact. From the villages, humans carried it into Africa's cities.

What of the Speckled Monster? Well, it **gave ground** slowly. Through vaccination, Sweden eliminated it first, in 1895, followed by Puerto Rico four years later. All the European countries eliminated it between 1920 and 1940. In the United States, the number of smallpox cases fell from 48,782 in 1930 to 9,877 in 1939 to eleven in 1951. From 1948 to 1965, the Speckled Monster took only one victim in the United States.

Despite these successes, smallpox still raged in other parts of the world because vaccination was not widespread enough to control it. In the twentieth century, this disease killed over 300 million people—three times the number of people who died in all the century's wars combined. In Asia, Africa, and Latin America, it took, on average, 5 million lives each year, every year. Although science now fights bacterial infections with drugs called antibiotics, these are useless against viruses, because viruses are not alive in the same way that bacteria are. They defeat the immune system differently. At best, doctors could make a smallpox sufferer comfortable while their immune system wrestled with the disease.

In 1966 the World Health Organization set out to annihilate smallpox for good. Led by an American, Dr. Donald A. Henderson, its Smallpox Eradication Program attacked with all the resources of modern science. Its method: mass use of vaccinia in **the target countries**. Teams of health workers vaccinated millions of people,

---

found its way into infected
gave ground went away
the target countries the countries that had smallpox

particularly children, always the **chief** victims. Yet results were disappointing. Despite their best efforts, the Speckled Monster continued to find victims. These were usually adults the vaccinators missed, or children born since the last mass vaccination. Would humanity ever conquer the disease?

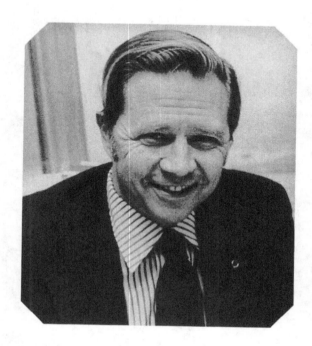

Dr. Donald A. Henderson led the campaign for the final conquest of smallpox in Africa. PHOTO COURTESY OF THE WORLD HEALTH ORGANIZATION

A New Approach to Vaccination Stops Smallpox

The answer came in the West African nation of Nigeria. In 1968 a vaccine shipment failed to arrive. That made smallpox researchers wonder if it was necessary to vaccinate every Nigerian. They decided to try a different approach.

....

chief main

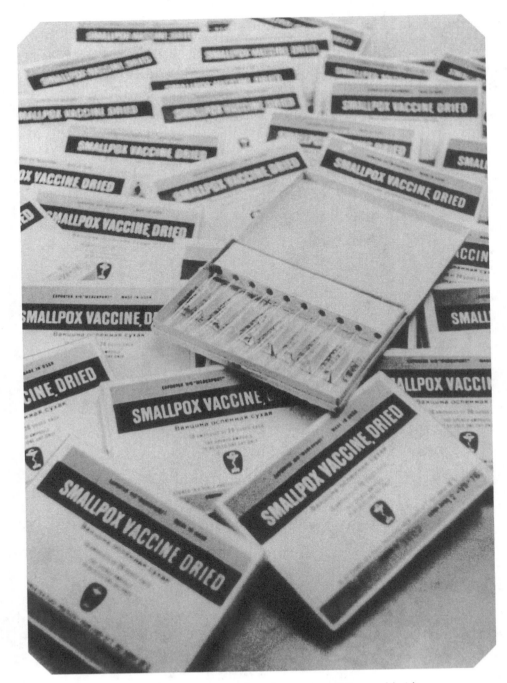

Millions of vaccine doses contributed to the success of the worldwide campaign to eradicate smallpox. PHOTO COURTESY OF THE WORLD HEALTH ORGANIZATION

Instead of mass vaccinations, they began a program of **"surveillance and containment."** The idea was to follow the Speckled Monster's every move. World Health Organization field-workers showed villagers pictures of babies covered with pustules. That way local people learned to recognize the disease and report cases quickly. The Nigerian authorities would then **cut the village off from the outside world** and have every villager vaccinated, or revaccinated. Their swift action killed the Speckled Monster wherever it reared its ugly head, keeping it from finding new victims. Scientists call this "breaking the chain of infection."

Thanks to surveillance and containment, the Speckled Monster disappeared from West and Central Africa by 1970. By 1975 it vanished from South America and Asia. In the fall of 1977, a cook named Ali Maow Maalin in the East African country of Somalia

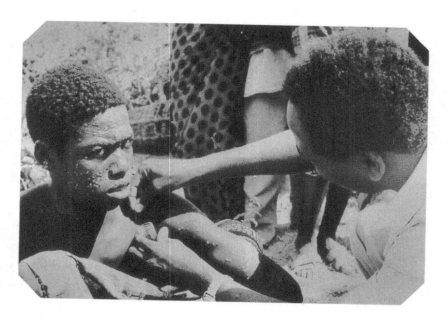

An essential part of eliminating smallpox in Africa was identifying the disease when it struck, isolating the victim's village, and vaccinating everyone in it. PHOTO COURTESY OF THE WORLD HEALTH ORGANIZATION

....

surveillance and containment watching for the disease and then stopping it by isolating infected people

cut the village off from the outside world isolate the village by not allowing anyone to enter or leave

became the last person to get the disease outside a laboratory setting. He survived. Smallpox took its last life in 1978. Janet Parker worked as a photographer in an English research laboratory. Somehow, the virus escaped from a container and infected her. She died from the disease. The World Health Organization declared final victory over smallpox the following year.

Victory ended smallpox vaccinations everywhere. No medical school graduate has seen a case of it for over twenty years. **Nowadays**, medical students read about the Speckled Monster as **a curiosity**, if at all. Edward Jenner's dream has come true. Smallpox is no more.

Or is it?

....

Nowadays Today
a curiosity an interesting story

BEFORE YOU MOVE ON...

1. **Problem and Solution** Reread page 89. Jenner's arm-to-arm method often spread other infections. How did doctors solve this problem?

2. **Cause and Effect** Reread pages 93–95. In 1968, vaccines did not arrive in Nigeria. How did this cause researchers to create a new system of vaccination?

LOOK AHEAD Do you think smallpox is gone forever? Read pages 98–105 to find out.

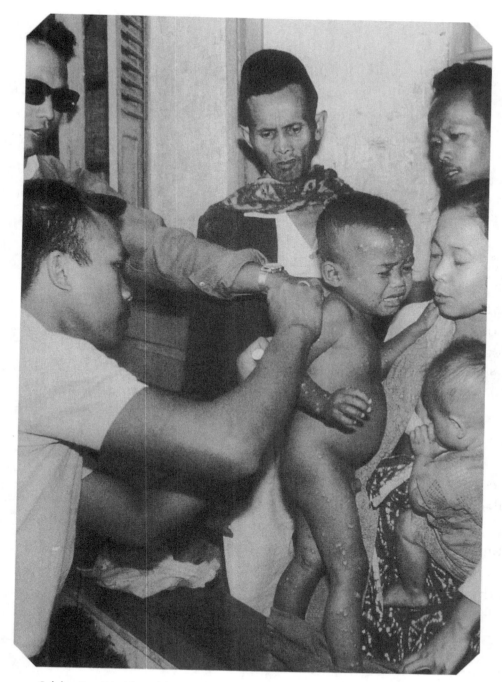

Celebrating World Health Day, 1975, with a mass vaccination of children in the Philippines. PHOTO COURTESY OF THE WORLD HEALTH ORGANIZATION

The *Frozen* Monster

Smallpox was used as
a weapon throughout history.

*T*he story of the Speckled Monster is not over. Scientists still keep variola to help them study other viruses, but mainly out of fear.

Smallpox has a long history as a weapon. Recall that it ravaged the Aztecs of Mexico in the early 1500s. Although the Spanish had not meant to cause an epidemic, other **colonizing forces** used it for just that. While fighting Native Americans in 1763, British general Lord Jeffrey Amherst asked an aide a question: "**Could it not be contrived to send the smallpox among those disaffected tribes of Indians?** We must, on this occasion, use every **stratagem to reduce them**."

The aide, Colonel Henry Bouquet, replied: "I will try to inoculate the Indians with some blankets that may fall into their hands and take care not to get the disease myself." The idea, he explained in another letter, was the Indians' "total extirpation"; that is, their total annihilation. Today we would say the British leaders meant to commit genocide, the planned extermination of an entire racial, ethnic, or national group. Colonel Bouquet sent the Indians blankets from a smallpox hospital as "peace offerings." The disease

---

colonizing forces conquering nations

Could it not be contrived to send the smallpox among those disaffected tribes of Indians? Can we plan to spread smallpox to rebellious Indian tribes?

stratagem to reduce them method to kill them

swept through the enemy tribes, weakening them and breaking their resistance to British rule.

Later, during the American Revolution, British officers left smallpox victims at likely campsites in order to infect George Washington's army. Washington, immune ever since he had the disease as a teenager, wrote the Massachusetts House of Representatives in December 1775: "The information I have received that the enemy intended spreading smallpox among us **I could not suppose them capable of**. I now must give some credit to it as it made its appearance on several of those who last came out of Boston." To avoid an epidemic, he ordered history's first mass inoculation. Early the next year, he had every soldier inoculated who had not had smallpox "in the natural way."

In the twentieth century, some military planners viewed variola as an acceptable weapon of mass destruction; that is, one that could kill millions of people in a very short time. During the Cold War, both American and Soviet laboratories developed means of growing and spreading the deadly virus. Variola can easily be grown in laboratories. Airplanes can spray it over wide areas as an aerosol—that is, a fine mist.

Why Smallpox Is Still a Threat

Oddly enough, the conquest of smallpox has in a certain way made it more dangerous than ever. Until his death, Jenner believed that cowpox vaccine gave lifelong protection. Yet even in his day, it had become clear that this was not so. Some vaccinated adults got smallpox

---

I could not suppose them capable of was very hard to believe

years later, and a few of these died. Jenner blamed these cases on "imperfect vaccination" with substances that seemed to be cowpox but were not. He was wrong. Within the last fifty years, researchers found that smallpox vaccinations do not give lifelong immunity; only surviving a bout with variola can do that. Scientists are not sure how long it takes for the protection given by vaccinia to wear off, only that it does. Perhaps the immune system "forgets" a vaccination with a virus only related to a variola.

Some scientists believe that vaccinated people begin to lose their resistance to variola after about ten years. For that reason, they need **booster shots**. Other scientists disagree; they believe that resistance may last up to thirty years. Clearly, more research is needed to learn whether and when, exactly, to give booster shots. To complicate matters further, a cowpox vaccination may **wear off faster** in one person than another, for reasons that are still unclear. Anyhow, all vaccinations against smallpox must eventually be renewed. In Jenner's day, milkmaids in daily contact with cows probably received their boosters naturally, without knowing it. The vaccinations Jenner gave James Phipps over the years also had the effect of booster shots.

In 1972 the United States stopped vaccinating for smallpox; the roughly 114 million Americans born since then, or 42 percent of the population, have never had a vaccination against the disease. On May 8, 1980, the World Health Organization (WHO) declared that science had eliminated smallpox everywhere. As a result, the rest of the world abandoned vaccination for smallpox. Since most past vaccinations probably now offer little if any protection, and no new vaccinations have been given for more than a generation, humanity may face a terrible crisis. Releasing the Speckled Monster would trigger a worldwide epidemic on the scale of the one that allowed

---

booster shots additional vaccinations
wear off faster not work as long

Cortés to conquer the Aztecs in 1521. Only today, the world's population is eight times larger than it was back then.

In 1976 the WHO also persuaded most countries to destroy the variola stocks they were using for research, or send them to the United States or Russia for safekeeping. Britain sent its stock to the United States. The other nations agreed to cook the virus in autoclaves—steel tanks containing superheated steam under pressure. Intense heat can destroy not only variola, but any virus. Nowadays, the U.S. Centers for Disease Control (CDC) keeps its variola at a laboratory in Atlanta, Georgia. Russia holds its variola at the State Research Institute of Virology and Biotechnology, **code-named** Vector, in Siberia. Until recently, the top-secret Vector laboratories did not appear on maps. Both nations have signed **treaties pledging themselves** not to use germ warfare.

In all, some six hundred plastic vials, each a half inch long, contain the world's last *known* stocks of variola. The vials stand upright in cardboard boxes on shelves in **padlocked** freezers, in locked rooms, guarded by soldiers. Their contents are frozen in liquid nitrogen at −94 degrees Fahrenheit. Those vials hold enough variola to infect every person on earth.

The WHO voted to destroy these stocks at a 1986 meeting and set December 31, 1993, as the deadline. That deadline came and went, but the vials remain in their freezers.

This is no accident. Instead, it is part of a continuing debate among scientists, political leaders, and the military. Those who favor destruction of the smallpox stocks argue that humanity must eradicate the Speckled Monster forever—and do it immediately. Their opponents admit that, so far, variola has never benefited humanity in any way. Yet they want to preserve it nevertheless. Continued study of

----

code-named known by the secret name
treaties pledging themselves agreements promising
padlocked securely locked

variola, they argue, may yield vital information in several areas. For example, can the study of variola help unlock the secrets of other viral diseases, like AIDS? Does variola have anything to teach us about the workings of the human immune system? Will having variola permit future scientists to study problems **undreamed of today**? Although nobody can answer these questions for sure, one thing is certain. Putting the last vials into the autoclaves will destroy variola forever—and with it any good that might come from studying it in the future.

Fear and distrust, however, are the main reasons for keeping variola. Governments worry that other governments, or even terrorist groups, may secretly be preparing to release disease-causing antigens against their enemies, especially smallpox. Peter Jahrling, an American scientist, explains: "I don't think there is any higher biological threat to this nation than smallpox. . . . If smallpox is outlawed, only outlaws will have smallpox." That is, if any country has cheated by hiding a supply of variola, or given it to terrorists, it could threaten the entire human race.

The senior George Bush, then U.S. president, had this in mind during the Persian Gulf War of 1991. The U.S. military told him it suspected Iraqi president Saddam Hussein of having variola and preparing to use it against Allied forces. **A ruthless tyrant, Hussein crushed uprisings of** his own people with poison gas in the 1980s, so the military knew he was capable of anything. President Bush warned that he would reply to Iraqi use of *any* disease-causing agent with "the utmost severity." Translation: Mr. Bush would drop nuclear bombs on Iraq. Apparently, the warning was taken seriously and these frightful weapons were not used.

....

undreamed of today no one has ever thought of

A ruthless tyrant, Hussein crushed uprisings of A cruel leader, Hussein stopped rebellions among

This helps explain why the World Health Organization's 1993 deadline came to nothing. New deadlines for the virus's destruction were set in 1994 and 1995. Again variola **won stays of execution as objectors**, including the U.S. government, expressed growing fears of a sneak attack. Finally, in May 1999, the WHO extended the stay until 2002. Meanwhile, in April 2001, the U.S. government ordered 40 million doses of smallpox vaccine—vaccinia—added to the 15.4 million doses it already had on hand. No official thinks these would be enough to halt an epidemic. Should anyone else release variola, the speed of modern transportation would quickly spread it around the globe.

The September 11, 2001, attacks on the World Trade Center in New York City and the Pentagon in Washington, D.C., **sent a shock wave of horror throughout** the world. It was bad enough that suicide hijackers crashed three airliners into these buildings, killing some 3,000 people. Soon after the attacks, a person or persons, still unknown, released through the mail the bacteria that cause anthrax, killing five Americans and infecting twelve others. Anthrax is caused when the bacteria release powerful toxins into the human body. The good news is that this disease is not contagious. You cannot get anthrax from another person, and it is treatable with antibiotics.

Smallpox is another matter. Since a virus causes it, antibiotics are useless: so far, smallpox is impossible to treat. Equally important, airplanes do not need to release variola as an aerosol to spread it. "Smallpox martyrs," people willing to die horribly for their cause, might have themselves infected with the virus to spread it. This seems unlikely, because an infected person would have to be very sick to spread the virus, which would probably **tip off** the authorities.

....

won stays of execution as objectors was not destroyed because the governments who complained

sent a shock wave of horror throughout terribly frightened

tip off alert

Yet we cannot afford to take chances, since **too much is at stake**. For that reason, in November 2001, President George W. Bush decided that the nation's remaining stocks of variola would not be destroyed in 2002. That would allow scientists to develop new smallpox vaccines and possible treatments, a process that may take years, possibly decades. The U.S. government also said that it knew of at least five countries that are violating the 1972 Biological and Toxin Weapons Convention barring these weapons of mass destruction. These are Iraq, North Korea, Iran, Libya, and Syria. Meeting in Geneva, Switzerland, World Health Organization officials agreed that smallpox still posed a serious threat. In January 2002, the WHO executive board ruled that the destruction of the last official stocks of variola be **postponed indefinitely**. "We regard the potential release of smallpox as a critical national and international issue," United States assistant surgeon general Kenneth Bernard told the board. "A case of smallpox anywhere is a case everywhere."

Meanwhile, the U.S. government announced it will produce not an additional 40 million doses of smallpox vaccine, but 209 million doses by the beginning of the year 2003. A French firm, Aventis Pasteur, has also promised to donate 75 million doses of smallpox vaccine it has stockpiled in Pennsylvania. What is more, scientists believe existing vaccine stocks can be diluted—cut—so that what used to be given as a single dose can be given to five people. However, poorer countries would find it much more difficult to get enough vaccine for their people than the United States.

Should an outbreak of smallpox occur in the United States, the government would probably not vaccinate the entire population. Instead, public health officials favor the surveillance and containment

....

too much is at stake there is too much to lose if the disease spreads again

postponed indefinitely delayed forever

method that worked so well in Africa during the 1960s and 1970s. Yet vaccination **is not foolproof**. Recent studies show that, in the past, for every million people vaccinated, about two died from the vaccine. This number would surely increase because of AIDS victims and others with weakened immune systems.

Our story, therefore, is not over. Nobody can tell what **the future holds**. However, this much is certain: Edward Jenner's cowpox experiments **held out the** hope that, by first conquering one disease, humanity might eventually conquer all diseases. Sadly, Jenner found no magical formula for conquering humanity's worst enemies—no scientist can. For fear, greed, anger, hatred, and stupidity **also belong to the human condition**. If the Speckled Monster should ever return, it will not mutate naturally from a farm animal. It will come from a vial in a laboratory freezer.

....

is not foolproof does not work every time

the future holds will happen

held out the gave people

also belong to the human condition are all human qualities

BEFORE YOU MOVE ON...

1. **Argument** Why do some people argue that the last stocks of smallpox vaccine should not be destroyed? Do you agree?

2. **Author's Point of View** Reread pages 104–105. How does the author feel about getting rid of smallpox? How do you know?

ndex

(Page numbers in *italics* refer to illustrations.)

*I*ndex, continued